Being A Woman

Your Questions Answered

DR GORDON TAN WEE TECK

To Dear Teary

With Best wishes

Dr Gordon Tan

SINGAPORE
OXFORD UNIVERSITY PRESS
1998

Dedication

To my dear wife and lovely children.

To womankind, especially all my patients. May you enjoy reading it as much as I have enjoyed writing it. It is also my sincere wish that your life and that of your loved ones be enriched by its contents.

Oxford University Press

Oxford   New York
Athens   Auckland   Bangkok   Bombay
Calcutta   Cape Town   Dar es Salaam   Delhi
Florence   Hong Kong   Istanbul   Karachi
Kuala Lumpur   Madras   Madrid   Melbourne
Mexico City   Nairobi   Paris   Singapore
Taipei   Tokyo   Toronto
and associated companies in
Berlin   Ibadan

Oxford is a trade mark of Oxford University Press

© *Oxford University Press 1998*
First published 1998

ISBN 0 19 588356 X

Printed by Kin Keong Printing Co. Pte. Ltd.,
Published by Oxford University Press Pte. Ltd.,
37 Jalan Pemimpin, #03-03 Union Industrial Building, Block A, Singapore 577177

Foreword

I am pleased to write a foreword to this informative book by Dr Gordon Tan. The book is aimed at women who may seek answers to many of the questions in relation to obstetrical and gynaecological problems. It is unique in that it is a compilation of questions and answers relating to Dr Tan's personal experiences as an obstetrician and gynaecologist and is therefore based on his own practice.

I am sure that many women will find it very helpful. It is in a format which is easy to read and would help women ask the appropriate questions when discussing their problems with their practitioners.

Naren Patel
President
Royal College of Obstetricians & Gynaecologists
London

Preface

The life of an obstetrician and gynaecologist is an interesting one. Helping women conceive, delivering babies, treating pelvic pain and infection, removing cysts and fibroids, receiving 'Thank You' cards and invitations to baby's first month celebrations all give me immense satisfaction. In the course of my day's work, my patients ask me many questions. Over the many years of my practice, I have compiled these questions into a book which would take a woman through from the time she takes her first breath until the time she bounces her own grandchildren on her knees.

This book is therefore unique. It is factual and informative, and is at times candid and irreverent. Most of all, it addresses my growing concern that many women either worry unnecessarily when there is no reason to, or do not worry when indeed they should. For example, the chapter *Waiting for Baby*, examines infertility, a problem which is often successfully treated just by simple measures and there is usually little cause for concern. On the other hand, the chapters *Sexually Transmitted Diseases (STDs) – Don'ts and More Don'ts* and *Serial Killers and Bumps in the Dark* highlight the potent dangers that lurk in certain behavioural attitudes. I hope that through reading these chapters, many women can avoid the tragedies I see in my practice.

This book is therefore something like life itself. It has the rough as well as the smooth, the light-hearted chapters like *With This Ring* and *The Happy Event* and the more serious ones like *Through the Scope* and *Under the Knife*, where gynaecological operations are discussed. Many patients have a tremendous fear of the unknown and to dispel these fears I have described the common gynaecological operations, some with the help of diagrams and photographs. I would like to express my gratitude to my many patients who have written the first-person accounts or have consented to photographs being taken of the various procedures.

While this book is enlightening, it is not my intention to make you a gynaecologist in three hours. As such, please consult your doctor when confronted with any of the conditions described.

Do take this book with you and read it at the hairdresser's or while waiting for your daughter's piano lesson to end. You will then have a better understanding of the various conditions that may afflict a woman and more importantly, appreciate the importance of prevention or the early detection of serious illnesses. *Being a Woman – Your Questions Answered* would then have achieved what it was designed to accomplish.

Dr Gordon Tan Wee Teck
1997

About the Author

Dr Gordon Tan Wee Teck graduated with the degrees of Bachelor of Medicine and Bachelor of Surgery in 1980. As an undergraduate, he obtained distinctions in biochemistry and microbiology and was awarded the Beecham book prize in microbiology in 1978.

Dr Tan sat for his post-graduate medical examinations in 1985. In the Master of Medicine (Obstetrics and Gynaecology) examinations, he was awarded the Fourth Asean Congress of Obstetrics and Gynaecology Gold Medal.

After his higher degree, Dr Tan had a short attachment with the Royal Northern and Islington Hospitals in London. He was admitted as a member of the Royal College of Obstetricians and Gynaecologists, London in 1986. In 1989, he was made a member of the Academy of Medicine, Singapore.

He has been in clinical practice since graduation and is currently a consultant obstetrician and gynaecologist at the Gleneagles and Mount Elizabeth Hospitals, Singapore.

Acknowledgements

My special thanks to the following people for their valuable comments and contributions to this book:

Blackwell Science Ltd
Food and Nutrition Department, Ministry of Health, Singapore

Dr Michael Adler, *Professor* in Genito-Urinary Medicine, The Middlesex Hospital, London

Dr Ang Chee Beng, *Consultant Dermatologist*, Mount Alvernia Medical Centre, Singapore

Dr R.D. Catterall, London

Dr Chan Heng Thye, *Consultant Orthopaedic Surgeon*, Gleneagles Medical Centre, Singapore

Dr Cheong Wai Kwong, *Consultant Dermatologist*, Specialist Centre, Singapore

Mr Richard Eu, LLB, *Chairman*, Eu Yan Sang Pte Ltd

Dr Goh Hak Su, *Consultant Colorectal Surgeon*, Gleneagles Medical Centre, Singapore

Dr Kwa Kie Tjong, *Consultant Anaesthetist*

Dr Charles Lacey M.D., Department of Genito Urinary Medicine, St. Mary's Hospital, London

Dr James Lee, *Orthopaedic Surgeon*, Gleneagles Medical Centre, Singapore

Dr Lim Kah Beng, *Consultant Dermatologist*, Gleneagles Medical Centre, Singapore

Dr Susan Lim, *Consultant Surgeon*, Gleneagles Medical Centre, Singapore

Dr Joanna Lin, *Oncologist*, Mount Elizabeth Medical Centre, Singapore

Dr Adrian Mindel, *Senior Lecturer* in Genito-Urinary Medicine, The Middlesex Hospital, London

Dr Ngiam Thye Eng, *Consultant Paediatrician*, Gleneagles Medical Centre, Singapore

Dr Ngoi Shing Shang, *Consultant Colorectal Surgeon*, Gleneagles Medical Centre, Singapore

Dr Tan Yew Oo, *Oncologist*, Mount Elizabeth Medical Centre, Singapore

Dr Tay Kah Phuan, *Urologist*, Gleneagles Medical Centre, Singapore

Dr William Yip, *Consultant Paediatrician*, Gleneagles Medical Centre, Singapore

Mrs Boon Oon San   )
Mrs Ivy Kwa   )   for their delicious recipes
Mrs Irene Tan Geok Gim)

Contents

- Cancer of the colon
- Breast cancer
- Lung cancer
- Ovarian cancer
- Cervical cancer
- Cancer of the endometrium
- Cancer of the vulva
- Bumping off the killers
- An apple (and more) a day ...
- How not to go up in smoke
- A hearty work-out
- De-stress or distress?

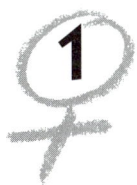

My Young Lady

What are little girls made of, made of?
What are little girls made of?
Sugar and spice and everything nice,
That's what little girls are made of, made of.

The newborn period and early childhood

Q What possible gynaecological problems can there be in a baby or preschool girl?

A The newborn usually enjoys good health. Protective antibodies, having crossed the placenta from the mother, protect the newborn from the common coughs and colds. Gynaecological conditions are generally rare but may sometimes occur. Among these conditions is the imperforate hymen.

Q What is an imperforate hymen?

A In some babies there is a membrane across the lower part of the vagina, usually just above the hymen. Above this obstruction, the vagina is distended by milky fluid. If a large quantity of fluid is present, the baby is irritable and cries excessively. The lower abdomen may be swollen and the baby may be unable to pass urine. Examination of the opening of the vagina (the vulva) of the baby usually shows a bulging membrane.

Q How is the imperforate hymen treated?

A The treatment for this condition is to make a simple cut in the membrane in order to release the retained fluid. This is done by a gynaecologist, with the patient under a short general anaesthesia.

Most cases of the imperforate hymen are detected either during the first week of life or not until the patient seeks medical attention for failing to menstruate at puberty.

The primary school years

Q What are the more common gynaecological conditions of the primary school years?

A The commonest problem during this period is infection of the opening and inner portions of the vagina (vulvovaginitis) by bacteria of low potency. Our tropical climate, with its high humidity, the relatively low levels of female hormones (oestrogens) in the child and the active school life which our children lead, all contribute to the development of this condition.

Q What does a child with vulvovaginitis complain of?

A She usually complains of itchiness of the vulva after a physically active day in school. Examination of the vulva would show mild swelling with redness. There would be a light yellowish to greenish discharge on the panties.

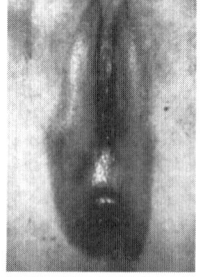

Vulvovaginitis

If the condition is more severe, she would then complain of vaginal soreness with pain on passing urine.

Q How is vulvovaginitis treated?

A Treatment is by the application of an oestrogen cream on the vulva every night for 2 weeks. This increases the natural resistance of the vagina and allows the body to overcome the non-specific infection. Over-the-counter antiseptics should not be used as these may cause chemical irritation, which usually makes matters worse.

Q Are there any other causes of vaginal discharge in a child?

A Sometimes a child would playfully insert a small object into her vagina. I have seen a small peanut, a pebble, a marble and even a small newspaper pellet! The child would complain of soreness of the vulva. The discharge in this instance is different from that in vulvovaginitis – this is more likely to be accompanied with blood stains and a foul odour. Upon direct questioning, the young child usually does not remember or may be too frightened to tell the truth. A simple examination under a light general anaesthesia would be necessary for removal of the object.

Q My daughter usually complains of itchiness around the anus and the opening of the vagina. There is just a little vaginal discharge. What could be the cause?

A In threadworm infection, the child complains more of itchiness in and around the anus and the vulva than of vaginal discharge. It is generally harmless but the usual medication for deworming, such as pyrantel pamoate, is recommended for persistent itching.

Q I have just noticed that the opening of my 6-year-old daughter's vagina has almost closed. Is this condition serious?

A In young girls, the lips of the entrance to the vagina (labia minora) sometimes fuse together almost overnight. This occurs from the back to the front, until only a small opening for passing urine remains. In treating this condition, the gynaecologist separates the labia using a fine probe and oestrogen cream is applied by the mother nightly. The adhesions then separate after about a week to 10 days.

Puberty and the teenage years

Q What are the first changes when a girl blossoms into a woman?

A Most mothers feel a twinge of sadness when their little baby girl shows signs of womanhood. The first changes are usually that of breast growth, which usually starts between the ages of 8 and 13 years. Breast growth begins with the development of the breast bud, which causes the nipple to enlarge and rise above the level of the surrounding breast. A spurt in height usually occurs at the same time and the young lady of the house suddenly discovers to her delight that she can strut convincingly in Mum's 3-inch heels!

Pubic hair growth usually follows and the development of underarm hair is next. This is in turn followed by the first menstrual period.

Over the last century, the age at which girls have their first menstruation (or menses) has been declining. Girls are reaching their first menstruation a year earlier than their mothers.

Q What causes menstruation?

A The diagram sums up the processes which bring about puberty and menstruation. The hormone control of menstruation begins in a part of the brain called the hypothalamus, which secretes substances called releasing hormones. These in turn act on another part of the brain called the pituitary gland, causing it to secrete two other hormones called follicular stimulating hormone (FSH) and luteinizing hormone (LH). FSH then acts on the ovaries, causing small bubbles called follicles to develop. Each follicle contains one egg or ovum. Of the many follicles, only one would enlarge and release the ovum when exposed to a surge of LH.

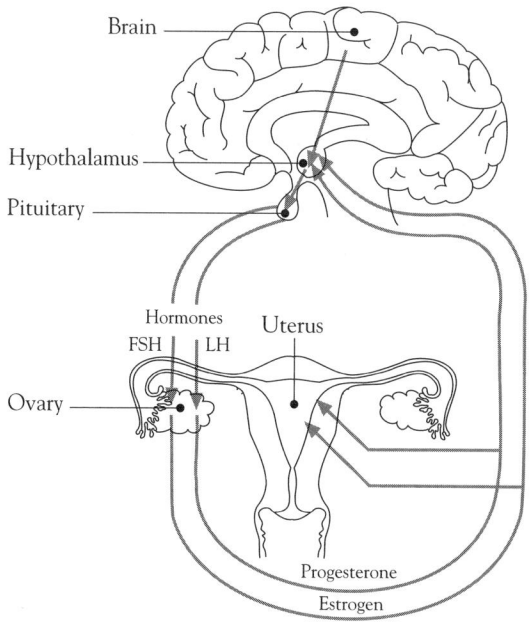

How puberty and menstruation comes about.

Development of the follicles results in the secretion of hormones called oestrogens. It is this gradual increase in oestrogen production and secretion as the child grows older that results first in the development of the breasts, pubic and underarm hair and the other female sexual characteristics, and later in the maturing of the womb and menstruation.

After the release of the ovum from the follicle (i.e. ovulation), the ovary secretes an additional hormone called progesterone. Both oestrogens and progesterone act on the lining of the womb to cause it to thicken. In the absence of pregnancy, the levels of oestrogens and progesterone fall and this brings on the onset of menstruation.

Why are menstrual problems common in the young adolescent?

Having seen the close interplay of the various hormones necessary for normal menstruation, we realize the ease with which problems in menstruation can occur. This is especially so during the first few years after the first menstruation as the cyclical production of the various hormones have yet to be established.

What are the more common menstrual problems in the young adolescent?

Not uncommonly, an anxious mother brings her daughter to consult me because her young adolescent has had no menstruation for a few months after the first menstruation. An examination of the young girl would reveal secondary sexual characteristics appropriate to her age. A rectal examination or a pelvic ultrasound would reveal a normal sized uterus. Both mother and daughter are then reassured that this lack of menstruation is due to the absence of ovulation, which is common during this phase of the young girl's life.

The problem usually resolves spontaneously, with the reappearance of the menstrual flow. It can also be brought on by a short course of oestrogens and progesterone if the menses has been absent for more than 6 months.

Sometimes the problem is that of heavy menstruation, which usually follows a period of a few months with no menstruation. Normal menstrual blood flow is dark red, with no blood clots or at most a few small clots. If the bleeding is heavy, a bright red colour or with large clots and especially when it is associated with dizziness, then the patient should seek medical attention.

Close questioning on the amount of blood lost would usually reveal the extent of the problem. The patient would be pale if the bleeding has been heavy. The size of the uterus is then checked using an ultrasound scanner or by a rectal examination. The latter is usually a shade uncomfortable for the patient. A simple blood test to determine the haemoglobin level is then done to determine the extent of the anaemia.

At this juncture, a wise doctor usually conducts a discreet pregnancy test for any disorder in bleeding, whether absent or excessive, even in girls whose virtue do not seem to be in question. I remember a plump 13-year-old schoolgirl in my early days as a doctor. She had had no menstruation for 7 months and had vehemently denied having any sexual contact. She was about to be sent to the pharmacy for some medication when I noticed the baby kicking through her baggy school uniform!

Q What is the treatment for heavy menstruation?

A For mild cases of heavy menstruation, it is usually sufficient to give firm reassurance to mother and child that such episodes are not uncommon and are usually transient. The patient is advised to eat a diet rich in iron and protein and is prescribed iron tablets. She is also asked to record on a calendar the days of menstrual bleeding and the days of light and heavy flow.

Heavy bleeding can be controlled with progesterone either in the form of an injection or tablets. Treatment is usually carried out by administering hormones for 3 months and then stopping all treatment. By that time, the normal cyclical hormonal profile would usually have been re-established.

If bleeding is so excessive that the patient suffers from dizzy spells, fainting or marked anaemia, then admission to hospital is necessary for more stringent tests and control of the bleeding.

Q What is the cause of painful menstruation and what does it actually feel like?

A This happens only in cycles where there is ovulation. Hence it is not a common problem in the first few months of menstruation when there is usually no release of any ovum from the ovaries. Later on, when the cycles become regular and ovulation occurs monthly, painful menstruation may become a troublesome condition.

The pain is classically a heaviness or a dull cramp in the lower abdomen and upper thighs, beginning a day before or during the first day of menstrual flow. The pain usually lessens with the onset of menstrual flow or on the following day. Menstrual pain almost always does not extend below the knees or above the navel. The pain may be severe enough to cause nausea, vomiting and even cold sweats and fainting.

Q What is the treatment for painful menstruation?

A General measures like exercises and warm baths usually help in mild cases. When the condition is severe, hot water bottles over the lower abdomen or medication with mefenamic acid from the day of the expected pain for 5 days would be necessary.

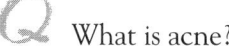

What is acne?

Pimples are extremely common at puberty in almost everyone, although they occur to different degrees. This problem usually improves in early adulthood. The common sites are the face, upper chest and back. When there are large numbers of pimples, the condition is referred to as acne.

What causes acne?

Acne is, to a large extent, inherited. If both parents had acne then the chances of their child developing acne at puberty is 50 per cent. At the time of puberty, small quantities of the male hormone testosterone are produced. It causes the sebaceous glands of the body, especially those on the face, to develop. These glands in turn secrete an oily compound called sebum. Bacteria in the sebaceous glands react with sebum and play a vital role in the development of acne.

In spite of the role of bacteria in the formation of pimples, this condition is not contagious.

In some patients, the acne worsens just before menstruation. This is due to the fall in the oestrogen levels before the onset of menstruation.

How is acne treated?

Acne vulgaris almost always heals spontaneously by early adulthood. Treatment, however, shortens the duration, reduces the severity of the disease and lessens complications such as scarring. In general, a clear skin boosts the self-image and improves the socialization of acne patients.

Q What is the role of skin cleansing?

A Acne is usually related to oily skin. Washing the face twice or three times daily with a glycerine soap is a useful way of removing excess surface grease. This can be followed by applying alcoholic preparations. It also helps to dab the skin lightly with grease-absorbing paper several times daily.

Q Does diet affect the severity of acne?

A Some parents consider certain foodstuffs as 'heaty' and believe that they aggravate pimple formation. The general diet, however, has no effect on sebum production, which is largely genetically predetermined. Hence it is not necessary to avoid favoured foods such as chocolates, curries, fried foodstuff, nuts or meats on this count. On the other hand, avoidance of such foods may not be a bad idea as obesity would cause a pimply teenager's already flagging morale to nosedive further.

However, iodides sometimes found in cough mixtures can aggravate inflamed pimples and should not be taken in large amounts.

Q What sort of psychological advice can we give to acne patients?

A Acne sufferers often suffer severely as a result of their skin condition. In fact, a lecturer once said, tongue-in-cheek, that one reason why the condition is called acne vulgaris is that the patients are often depressed to the point of being vulgar! Withdrawal, feelings of anxiety and depression are common reactive responses. Acne is, however, not the result of mental factors. Acne treatment therefore rests primarily on active drugs and not psychotherapy. Psychotherapy, if used, supplements drug therapy by boosting optimism and treatment compliance in a disease where medication is usually tedious and long-term. This therapy includes the build-up of self-worth and the reinforcement of positive factors in the patient's physical attributes.

Q Which drugs are often used in the treatment of acne?

A This varies with the form of acne. The most active form of treatment is a peel to eliminate the blackheads and whiteheads (comedones) and prevent their recurrence. The treatment can be given in the form of a solution, cream or gel of vitamin A acid. The side-effects include redness, scaling, itching or at worst, a temporary worsening of the condition at the beginning of the treatment. The patient should take heart as these side-effects, although unavoidable, are only temporary.

Another effective peeling agent which also kills bacteria is 3, 5 or 10% benzoyl peroxide in gel form.

In mild cases or in patients with especially sensitive skin, frequent cleansing with hypoallergenic soap solutions or glycerine soaps is recommended. Camouflage lotions or creams can then be used for big social occasions. A few small blackheads or whiteheads can be individually removed with a comedo extractor, following moist compresses and hot face masks.

Extreme care must, however, be taken especially for closed blackheads and for pimples around the centre of the face as infection in this area can have serious consequences. Such infections may travel backwards via connecting vessels to a structure at the base of the brain called the cavernous sinus. Spread of infection to this area may lead to fits, coma and even death.

Q   My teenage daughter has large pimples on her face which contain pus. How can this condition be treated?

A   In patients with inflamed pimples containing pus, careful skin cleansing is again necessary. Peeling treatment is then carried out with vitamin A acid or benzoyl peroxide preparations. If the pimples contain pus, then antibiotics are used either directly on the pimples in the form of tetracycline or erythromycin creams or ointments, or tetracycline or erythromycin capsules taken orally. Treatment begins with high doses until there is significant improvement, which may be apparent only after a few weeks. Thereafter, the antibiotics are given over a few months or until the acne clears up.

Q   How can we treat the severe form of acne which produces large lumps?

A   Some patients develop a very severe form of acne in which the individual pimples become large and swollen and appear as lumps on the face. For this condition, treatment involves giving it the whole works, i.e. soaps and peeling agents, direct application and high-dose oral tetracycline or erythromycin antibiotics. Sometimes, hospital treatment may be required as there may be complications associated with the use of high-dose antibiotics. Larger lumps containing blood or pus are drained by a qualified doctor using large-bore needles under strict aseptic conditions. If this is unsuccessful, then tiny incisions are made using a lancet or small scalpel. In large bumps which contain no blood or pus, injections with a crystalline suspension of corticosteroid is used and this produces notable results in a few days, when the lumps flatten and regress.

Q Is any new drug available for acne treatment?

A A drug called isoretinoin can be given on its own. After 12 to 20 weeks, the patient is usually free of acne and remains so for many years. However, side-effects are not uncommon and these include dryness of the skin and lips, muscle aches and rise in blood cholesterol levels. This drug is used mainly in severe disfiguring acne that does not respond to standard treatment. As it can cause abnormalities to a growing fetus, it must not be used in pregnant women or for those who wish to conceive.

For women with no contra-indications, I usually prescribe contraceptive preparations containing oestrogens or a combination of cyproterone acetate and ethinyl estradiol, which causes most acne conditions to regress. However, treatment may last for many months.

Q How can the scarring from prolonged acne be treated?

A After long periods of treatment, the acne reaches a 'burnt out' state, sometimes with considerable scarring. This is then treated by a competent dermatologist or plastic surgeon who performs dermabrasion or excision of crater-like scars.

Q Are abdominal lumps common in young girls?

A Fortunately, abdominal lumps are uncommon in young girls and cancer of the reproductive organs even rarer.

Q What are common growths of the reproductive organs in young girls?

A The commonest ovarian tumour in the child and the adolescent is a benign growth called the teratoma or dermoid cyst. The patient usually complains of low abdominal pain. With larger cysts, the abdomen may be swollen. An X-ray of the abdomen would usually show deposits of calcium and this virtually confirms the diagnosis of a dermoid cyst.

Treatment of this condition is surgical. With the patient under general anaesthesia, the cyst can be removed with a laparoscope. The patient can then go home the same day.

Q Does cancer occur in this age group?

A Sarcoma botryoides is a rare cancer of the genital tract. The patient suffers from excessive discharge or irregular bleeding. Examination shows a grape-like growth arising from the walls of the vagina or the cervix. This rare and highly malignant tumour is treated by using a combination of chemotherapy and extensive surgery.

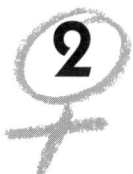

2

With This Ring ...

'Dear, I really love you and want to spend the rest of my life with you, but before we do that could you tell me your ABO blood group and Rhesus status please?'

Choosing a spouse

Life used to be simple when love was the only consideration in choosing a spouse. Then came the five Cs – Career, Cash, Credit card, Condominium and Car. Is there a sixth – Consanguinity or Compatibility of blood groups?

On a few occasions, I have had a young woman come in tearfully to my clinic lamenting, 'I'm in love with him but he's also a Lim' or 'I really love my fiancee but we have the same blood group.'

Q Does marriage between relatives lead to abnormal children?

A It is well known that marriage between two close relatives increases the risk of having abnormal babies, owing to the expression of recessive genes in the family. However, sharing the same surname is generally safe as long as the couple is not closely related.

Q What do you mean by a recessive gene and when does it 'express' itself?

A Genes are the materials which pass characteristics on from parent to child and they usually come in pairs. For each pair of genes you have, one is from your father and the other is from your mother.

Also, given a pair of genes, one could be normal and the other abnormal. The abnormal gene in this pair is said to be recessive if the person does not suffer from the abnormal condition. Only when the child inherits a pair of recessive genes, one from each parent, does he suffer from the abnormal condition.

Q What are blood groups?

A The blood in each individual person is unique in that it can be classified into various different blood groups. However, the two most important groups for practical reasons are the ABO and Rhesus blood groups.

Q What is the significance of the ABO and Rhesus blood groups in having babies?

A The ABO grouping is important for purposes of blood transfusion and has no bearing whatsoever in a person's reproductive status as well as the quality of the offspring.

The Rhesus group is, however, more significant for child-bearing. A person is either Rhesus-positive or Rhesus-negative. Less than 1 per cent of our local population is Rhesus-negative and it is this group which has the potential for problems. Should a Rhesus-negative woman marry a Rhesus-positive man, the first pregnancy would pose no problems.

However, in the course of the first pregnancy or the delivery, if the baby is Rhesus-positive, then blood from the baby may cross into the mother's blood stream to sensitize the mother. This leads to the production of anti-Rhesus antibodies in the mother. In the second or subsequent pregnancies, if the fetus is again Rhesus-positive, these anti-Rhesus antibodies would cross the placenta and destroy the red blood cells of the fetus, causing marked anaemia, generalized swelling, heart failure and eventual death of the fetus (hydrops fetalis).

Q Can this condition be prevented?

A This condition can, however, be prevented by injecting the mother with a drug called Rhogam immediately after the delivery of a Rhesus-positive baby. This prevents the sensitization and the subsequent production of anti-Rhesus antibodies in the mother.

Q Is a person's general health important if pregnancy is desired?

A At the marriage or pre-pregnancy consultation, enquiries are made on the patient's general health, with particular attention given to diseases like diabetes, hypertension and asthma. A family history of these diseases is significant as it predisposes the patient to developing these diseases later. Should these diseases already exist, then they should be treated prior to pregnancy to minimize the development of complications later.

Q What is beta thalassaemia?

A This is an inherited blood disorder which is relatively common. Approximately 1 to 2 per cent of the population are carriers of beta thalassaemia. These carriers lead perfectly normal lives and are normal in every respect except for having a slightly lower blood count (anaemia).

However, problems would arise when two beta thalassaemia carriers marry. The couple would then have a 1 in 4 chance of having a baby severely affected by the disease (beta thalassaemia major). In this condition, there is excessive breakdown of red blood cells, releasing iron pigments which are deposited in vital organs like the heart and liver. The patient usually dies in their late teens or early twenties. The couple would have a 1 in 2 chance of producing a child who is another beta thalassaemia carrier and another 1 in 4 chance of producing a perfectly normal child who is not a carrier of beta thalassaemia.

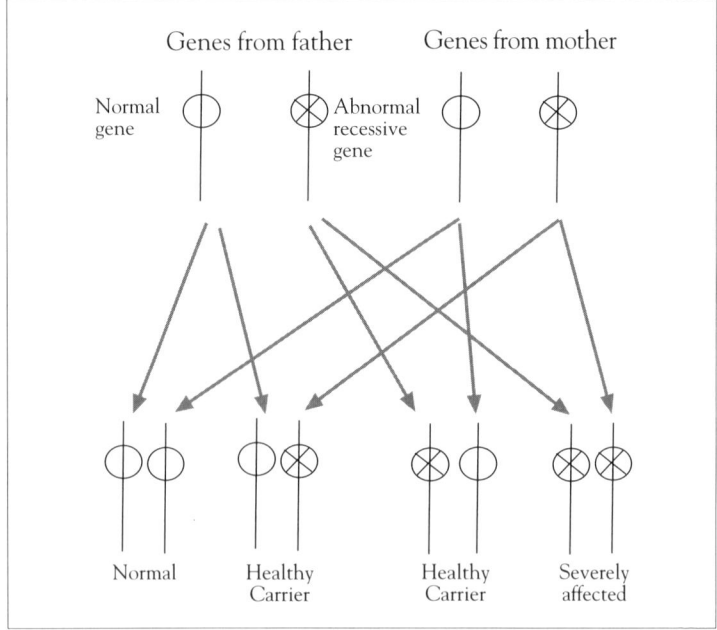

How a recessive gene is passed on from parents to children.

Q What about alpha thalassaemia?

A This is another inherited blood disorder with a carrier incidence of approximately 1 per cent in the general population. Like beta thalassaemia, carriers of alpha thalassaemia are generally healthy except for mild anaemia. The inheritance of this disease is slightly more complex than that for beta thalassaemia. Generally two healthy carriers have a 1 in 4 chance of having a fetus severely affected by alpha thalassaemia. The fetus has severe anaemia and does not survive until birth. It dies in the womb sometime in the course of the pregnancy. The fetus is extremely bloated from the heart failure which results from severe anaemia and is given the term 'hydrops fetalis'. The chances of the couple having a normal baby is 1 in 4 and that of them giving birth to a healthy carrier is 1 in 2.

Q So what happens when an alpha thalassaemia carrier marries a beta thalassaemia carrier?

A Strangely enough, the worst that happens is a 1 in 4 chance of having a child with mild anaemia. They have a 1 in 2 chance of producing either an alpha or a beta thalassaemia carrier and a 1 in 4 chance of having a perfectly normal child.

Q Is intelligence inherited?

A When a couple marries and starts a family, they would naturally want to have bright high-achieving children. In choosing a spouse, a man or a woman might also wonder whether their intelligence would be inherited.

Mr and Mrs Ang are two Fulbright scholars who realize to their horror that junior is only half-bright. 'What on earth happened to you? We used to get straight As in school and you only get Bs. No more TV and violin lessons. We're getting you extra tuition!'

In another neighbourhood many down-market kilometres away, Ah Chye's illiterate mother proudly proclaims to his aunt, 'Ah Chye chin kiang. Jip twa oak.' (Ah Chye is very bright. He made it to the University).

Both the jubilant Ah Chye (celebrating his A-levels success in the noisy neighbourhood restaurant), and the dumbfounded junior Ang (stewing in his bedroom), do not realize that they are actually fulfilling a very well-known phenomenon in life briefly summed up as 'nature tends to preserve the norm'.

What this means is that when two brilliant beings come together, their children are usually bright but not as brilliant as their parents and when two less intelligent beings marry, their children tend to be more intelligent than their parents. This is so that the normal distribution or bell-shaped curve for intelligence in the following figure is preserved.

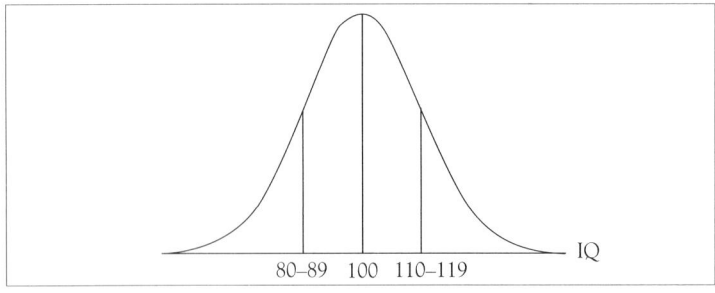

Notice how the IQ of the bulk of the population falls into the middle range.

If the children of bright parents were always bright and those of less intelligent parents even duller, then in time to come we would end up with two groups of people – one very bright and the other very dull, which is obviously not the case.

Infectious diseases and pregnancy

Q   What is measles? Are there different types?

A   Yes, the different types are German measles, 'true measles' and 'false measles'. The nature and significance of these conditions also differ.

Q   Is German measles (rubella) dangerous in pregnancy?

A   This is a disease of great significance to the woman who intends to have a baby. This is because infection during pregnancy, especially the first 12 weeks, would cause severe fetal malformations in 25 to 40 per cent of cases.

Q   What are the symptoms of German measles?

A   Rubella is a common disease of childhood caused by a virus. After an incubation period of 14 to 21 days, mild symptoms like a running nose and a low-grade fever appear. The most characteristic sign is the enlargement of lymph nodes behind the ears, neck and back of the head. These appear as small rubbery lumps the size of marbles and are painful when pressed. Discrete red spots appear on the roof of the mouth. A day after the appearance of the swollen lymph nodes, a rash develops. It appears on the face and spreads quickly to the body. The patient may complain of mild itching. The rash usually clears by the third day and the fever subsides. Unlike true measles, German measles does not cause the patient to be uncomfortable in the presence of bright lights.

Q Can a woman catch German measles a second time?

A Most women would be immune to German measles, having either caught the disease in childhood or been immunized at Primary Six. There is, however, a 5 per cent chance of a woman contracting rubella a second time after a natural infection. This would depend on the level of her protective antibodies and the strength of the viral contact. The incidence of infection following a vaccine is higher, in the region of 8 per cent. Hence it is usually advisable to get a booster vaccine 3 months before a woman intends to start a family.

Q What if a woman becomes pregnant soon after a German measles vaccination?

A Sometimes a patient discovers that she is pregnant within 3 months of a rubella vaccination and fears that the baby would be born abnormal. Although the rubella vaccine is that of a live virus, the virus has been so severely treated as to have lost all its 'teeth'. Studies have shown that babies born to such mothers have no increased incidence of abnormalities although the virus could be isolated from some of the newborn.

Q What is true measles (rubeola)?

A This is a highly contagious disease characterized by three stages. First, there is an incubation period of 10 to 12 days. Next, white spots appear in the mouth or throat. Finally, a rash appears successively over the neck, face, body, arms and legs, accompanied by a high fever. During this stage, the patient is more ill than the patient with German measles.

Complications are also more common than in German measles. These include infections of the ear (otitis media), lungs (pneumonia) and even the brain (encephalitis). Deaths from true measles are more common than from German measles but these are now fortunately rare, owing to the compulsory administration of the measles–mumps–rubella (MMR) vaccination in childhood.

Q What is false measles (roseola infantum)?

A This is as acute viral disease of infants and young children. The onset is sudden, with a fever which rises abruptly to between 39 and 40°C. The throat may be slightly inflamed but characteristically there is very little to explain the high fever. After 3 to 4 days, when the parents are at their wits' end, a rash appears on the child's body. It begins on the trunk, spreading mainly to the arms and neck. Little of it appears on the face and legs. This distinguishes it from the rash of rubella and rubeola.

The fever subsides when the rash appears. Other than the occasional fit from the high fever or dehydration, complications are rare.

Of the three, only rubella or German measles is of significance as far as pregnancies are concerned.

Q What is syphilis?

A Another condition to look out for during the pre-marriage consultation is syphilis. This is detected through a blood test called the VDRL in an asymptomatic patient. Should this be positive, then a further, more specific test called the TPHA is carried out to confirm the diagnosis. Although rare nowadays, syphilis should be aggressively treated as it can lead to stillbirths and severe malformations in the newborn.

Q How will I know if I have a vaginal infection?

A This may sometimes be present in patients with no symptoms although excessive vaginal discharge or itchiness around the genital region are the more common complaints.

Q What are the common causes of vaginal infections?

A In the tropics, thrush or candidiasis is the most common cause of excessive discharge and itchiness. The second most common cause is infection with a parasite known as *Trichomonas*. A painless vaginal swab and laboratory examination would confirm the diagnosis. Thrush is treated with an antifungicide which comes in the form of a tablet called a pessary. The pessary is inserted into the vagina. Oral tablets of metronidazole are given for *Trichomonas* infections.

Q What is a Pap smear?

A This is a screening test for cervical cancer and is performed on any patient who has been sexually active. Cervical cancer tends to occur in younger women who have multiple sexual partners or who began sex at an early age and in women who smoke. The real value of the Pap smear is that it can actually detect precancerous cells so that treatment can be started before the development of overt cancer.

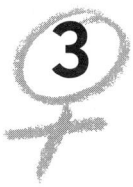

3 Waiting for Baby

'Familiarity breeds contempt – and children.'
            Mark Twain (1835–1910) in Notebooks, 1935
For many couples who work at it, Mark Twain is only half right.
Familiarity breeds love. For yet other couples who also work at it,
he is all wrong. Familiarity does breed love, but babies take a long
time to come.

How a new life begins

Q How are babies formed?

A Every month, one egg develops within one of the ovaries in the woman. The first day of the menstrual flow is day 1 of the menstrual cycle. Around day 14 of the cycle, a hormone (luteinizing hormone or LH) from the pituitary gland in the brain causes the egg to be released from the ovary. This egg then finds its way to the end of the Fallopian tube as shown in the figure on the following page.

During sexual intercourse, semen is deposited in the vagina. Sperms swim up the cervix through the top of the womb into the Fallopian tube.

Upon entering the Fallopian tube, the egg moves along and meets the sperm at approximately a third of the way down the tube. Conception then occurs with the egg fusing with the sperm to form the embryo. This usually occurs around day 16 or 17 of the menstrual cycle.

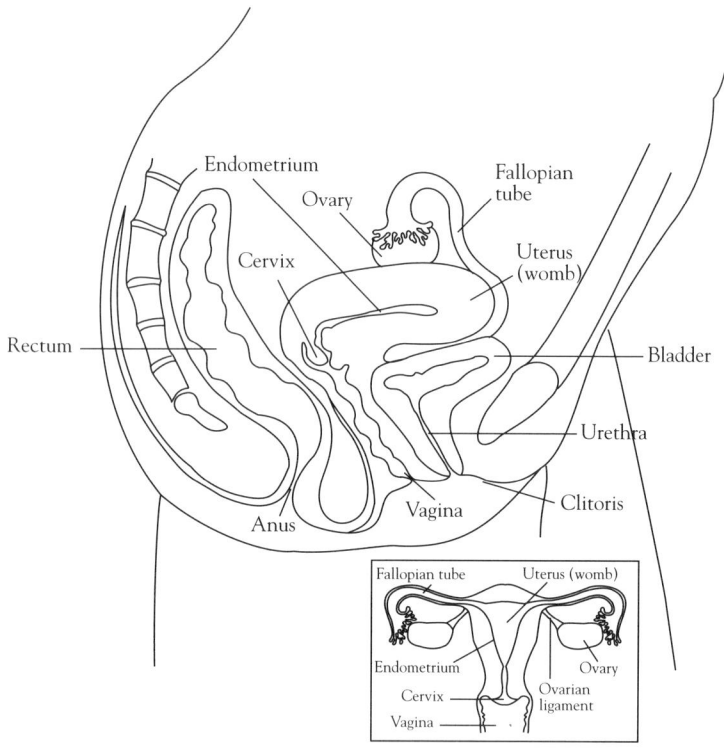

The female reproductive system

The embryo then tumbles along the remaining two-thirds of the Fallopian tube and enters the womb around day 20 of the cycle. The embryo then attaches and buries itself into the wall of the womb on day 21 of the cycle. By now, the embryo would have formed a bag of fluid around itself commonly called the water bag (the gestational sac). The embryo continues to grow into the wall of the womb until the 12th week.

Usually a pregnancy is diagnosed 2 weeks after a missed period with a urine test. By that time, 6 weeks from the first day of the last menses, the embryo would be about 4 mm in length. However, even though small, most of the major organs such as the heart, lungs and limbs would be almost formed. It is important to note this because any possible harm to the fetus, for example, through exposure to X-rays, would have occurred even before the woman realizes that she is pregnant.

Q How are sperms and semen formed?

A Sperms (spermatozoa) are formed in cells of the testes at the time of the male puberty. The sperms are then stored in an organ called the epididymis which is located in the upper part of the testes. The diagram on the following page clarifies this.

Semen is the fluid which is produced by the seminal vesicles and prostate gland in the male. It is greyish white, alkaline and contains fructose. The alkaline medium of semen counteracts the acidity of the vagina and is important for sperm survival, while fructose is a sugar which provides nutrition for the sperms.

Q What is ejaculation?

A In the male, during the climax of sexual intercourse, sperms and seminal fluid travel through the vas deferens and through the penis. The ejaculate is greyish and is released as a series of spurts, owing to the rhythmic contractions of the muscles of the penis. Each ejaculation releases about 2 to 4 cc of seminal fluid, which contains between 40 and 60 million sperms per cc! There are actually enough sperms in the normal ejaculate to create 240 million babies!

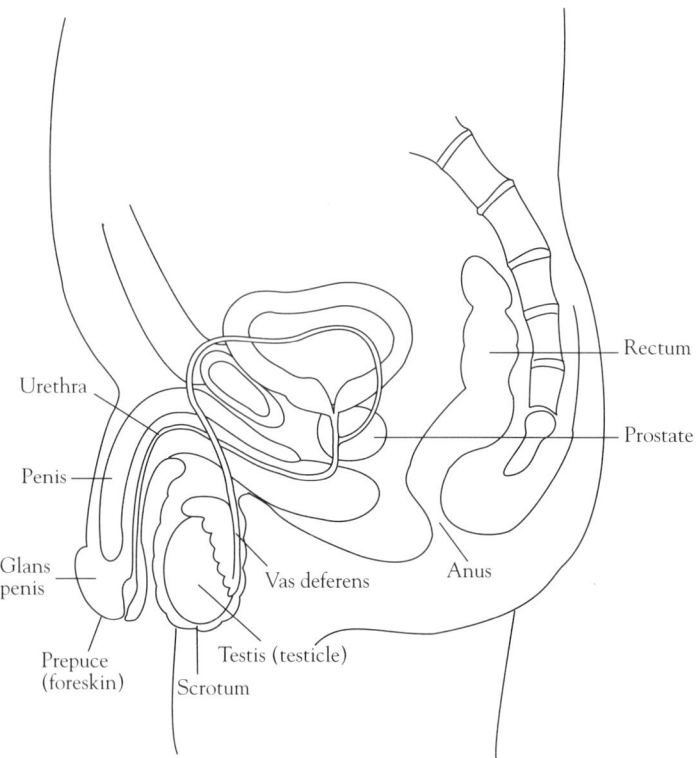

Urethra

Penis

Glans
penis

Prepuce
(foreskin)

Scrotum

Testis (testicle)

Vas deferens

Anus

Prostate

Rectum

The male reproductive system

Infertility

Q What is infertility?

A Infertility is the inability to have children. Normally, 90 per cent of healthy couples would be able to conceive after a year of trying.

Needless to say, infertility is an extremely distressing situation for the couple. However, the good news is that in many instances, simple measures are all that is required for pregnancy to occur.

Q Is infertility a serious problem?

A No, it usually is not. In my experience, most cases of infertility are quite easy to cure without the need for expensive and painful operations.

Q What are the common causes of infertility?

A Infertility can be attributed to female factors (70 per cent), male factors (20 per cent) and unknown factors (10 per cent). The following table summarizes and breaks down these causes.

Of the female factors, the commonest is endometriosis, the failure to produce eggs (anovulation), blocked Fallopian tubes and problems with hormone production after the release of the egg (luteal phase defects). Problems with the womb and its lower opening (the cervix) make up the remainder of the causes of infertility in women.

Causes of infertility

Female factors	
• Endometriosis	23%
• Failure to produce eggs	20%
• Problems with the tubes	15%
• Poor hormone secretion by the ovaries	7%
• Problems with the womb	5%
Male factors	20%
Unknown causes	10%

Endometriosis

Q What is endometriosis?

A Endometriosis is a disease in which the inner lining of the womb is found in places outside the womb. This usually occurs in the ovary or in the lower part of the abdomen just outside the womb.

Q How do I know if I have endometriosis?

A There are varying degrees of severity for this condition. The vast majority of women with endometriosis do not even know they have this condition as it is very mild (minimal endometriosis). Others complain of painful menstruation, pain during intercourse and even bleeding when passing motion during menstruation if the endometriosis is found in the rectum.

Endometriosis of the ovaries often occurs as a collection of blood in a thin-walled capsule (the endometriotic cyst or blood cyst). The woman would then complain of low abdominal pain, usually on one side, which gets worse during the menstruation. If this cyst is large, then she may notice a swelling of the lower abdomen or that her clothes have become too tight.

I have removed an endometriotic cyst the size of a football from a 23-year-old woman!

Q Who usually gets endometriosis?

A Any woman in the reproductive age can suffer from endometriosis – even those who are unmarried and those with many children. However, this condition is more common in busy working executives who delay having children.

Q How can we treat endometriosis?

A For mild cases or when there are small blood cysts, treatment with medication is usually effective. This takes the form of oral tablets of danazol to be taken daily for 6 to 8 months. Alternatively, a hormone preparation called a GnRH analogue may be used. This medication can be inhaled through the nose twice a day for 6 to 8 months or be given through monthly injections, again for 6 to 8 months.

For more serious cases of endometriosis, an operation is required.

Q Are there any side-effects from these medications?

A Yes, treatment with danazol can cause pimples, increase in facial hair or even hoarseness of the voice. GnRH analogue treatment may cause hot flushes like those of the menopause, dryness of the vagina or thinning of the bones. Also, while the patient is under GnRH analogue treatment, she is unable to get pregnant.

Q What sort of operation is done for more serious forms of endometriosis? Is it painful?

A Surgical treatment for endometriosis usually takes the form of laparoscopy. The patient is first placed under general anaesthesia so that no pain is felt. A needle is inserted into the navel to inflate the abdomen with carbon dioxide gas. When the abdomen is sufficiently distended, a metal tube (the laparoscope) is then inserted. The laparoscope enables the surgeon to see the internal organs. Two smaller instruments as shown in the second photograph below are then inserted lower down and the surgeon uses these like 'chopsticks' to remove diseased tissue. Endometriotic cysts of the ovaries can thus be removed. Smaller deposits of endometriosis the size of match-heads can be burnt using laser. Sometimes, when endometriosis has been present for a long period, the internal organs can be stuck together by scar tissue. This can also be cleared using laser.

The Fallopian tubes are then checked by pumping a blue dye through to see whether there is any blockage of the tubes which would prevent pregnancy. After the operation, the gas is released from the abdomen and each of the small punctures in the skin closed with a small stitch.

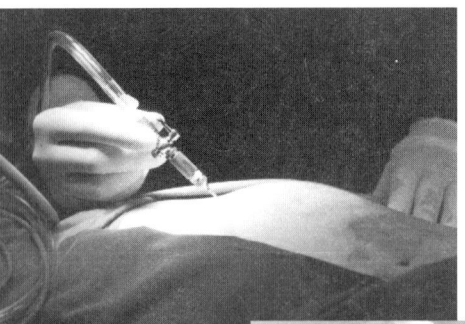

Gas is introduced into the abdomen to prepare for laparoscopic surgery.

With a laparoscope in one hand and surgical forceps in the other, the surgeon removes the cyst.

How long do I need to stay in hospital after laparoscopic surgery?

In most instances, the patient is discharged the very same day. Here is a first-person account of a patient who underwent laparoscopic surgery:

When my gynaecologist diagnosed a 5-cm cyst in my right ovary, I was very worried. I was admitted at 9 a.m. for the laparoscopic operation which was scheduled at 2 p.m. the same day. I had only taken a light breakfast at 8 a.m. As I waited in the ward, I wondered whether the butterflies in my stomach were due to hunger or anxiety.

A cheerful nurse then came into the room and told me to remove my jewellery, false teeth (thank God I had none!) and contact lenses. She then wiped off my lipstick, removed my nail polish and gave me a gown to change into. She asked me to lie down and then shaved the lower part of my abdomen.

Next, an attendant wheeled in a trolley. At the sight of the trolley, the butterflies in my stomach did somersaults! I was then wheeled into the operating theatre. The lights were very bright and the place smelled slightly fragrant. What I did not expect was the laughter and noise and the sight of everybody dressed in green. Everyone was relaxed and made the operating room appear like any other place. The butterflies in my stomach settled.

My gynaecologist reassured me that all would be fine. Soon another blue-capped doctor appeared and introduced himself as the anaesthetist. After asking me about drug allergies and giving me reassurance, he told me that he was going to insert a drip in my left hand. He then slapped my left hand (which reminded me of what my teacher did during my naughty schooldays) and gave me a local pain-relieving injection which felt like an ant bite. After the drip was inserted, I tried to keep my eyes open but could not. I then saw a red and a green light.

The next thing I knew, someone was slapping my face and saying, 'Operation's over. Wake up. Wake up.' I felt something in my throat which made me want to cough and I saw a bright light above me. I felt no pain, only dizziness, and dozed off again. When next I awoke, I was in my hospital bed. My stomach and neck felt sore, as if I had had an hour of vigorous aerobics. Other than that, I felt rather fine. My gynaecologist then appeared with a nurse and showed me what he had removed in a bottle. That almost made me feel sick again, but I was extremely relieved when he told me that the operation was a success and that the cyst was not cancerous.

I went home at 8 p.m. the same day. I felt slightly sore in the throat and over the belly the following day but was able to potter around the house and even cook for my husband!

Q Can endometriosis be prevented?

A Endometriosis is a disease of the fertile years. Hence it tends to improve after menopause. Having children is a good way to minimize the extent of the disease. There is no specific food which prevents the disease.

Failure to produce eggs

Q How do I know that I am producing eggs every month?

A A woman who is ovulating monthly usually has regular menstruation lasting 2 to 7 days, at intervals of 25 to 32 days. There is often low abdominal pain during the first 2 days of menstruation.

During the time when the egg is released, which is usually between day 12 and day 16 from the first day of the menstruation, a woman is likely to experience the following symptoms:

- clear vaginal discharge which is stringy like egg-white,
- a dull ache in the lower tummy, usually on one side
- slight bleeding from the vagina which lasts one day
- tenderness of the breasts

Taking the temperature daily using a special thermometer will show a slight rise in temperature during the second half of the menstrual cycle if there is ovulation.

Q What medication is there to help egg production?

A Oral tablets called clomiphene can be given from day 3 to day 7 of the menstrual cycle. These are given in increasing doses every month until ovulation or pregnancy occurs. In patients who do not produce eggs even with clomiphene, a stronger drug comprising follicular stimulating hormone (FSH) and luteinizing hormone (LH) is given through daily injections. Close medical supervision with ultrasound scans and blood tests are needed to prevent complications. When the ultrasound scan shows that the egg is 'ripe' then another injection containing human chorionic gonadotrophin (HCG) is given to bring about actual release of the egg from the ovary. A third drug which is also used is gonadotrophin releasing hormone (GnRH). This drug is put in a portable automatic infusion pump and delivered through a needle under the skin. The patient carries this with her wherever she goes. Again, medical supervision is required to avoid complications as the dosage of the drug needs to be carefully monitored.

Q Are there any side-effects with these drugs?

A Clomiphene causes twins in 5 per cent of patients. Importantly, birth defects are not more common in patients taking clomiphene. It has been suggested that high doses of the drug increases the risk of miscarriages and enlargement of the ovaries but this has not been proven.

Side-effects with FSH treatment can be more serious. Fever may sometimes occur. If not carefully monitored, the ovaries may swell into big cysts. When this happens, the patients may even need to be hospitalized. In rare instances, an operation may be needed to treat these complicated cysts.

GnRH treatment via the infusion pump causes hot flushes, irritability and sometimes infection where the needle is inserted into the skin.

Q What is the cervix? Has it a role to play in infertility?

A The cervix is the lower portion or the neck of the womb. It acts as a biological valve which allows sperms to enter the womb at certain periods of the menstrual cycle and blocks their entry at other times. The cells of the cervix produce a thin clear mucus during the time the egg is released and this clear mucus allows the sperms to pass through. After this fertile period, the cells produce thick mucus which blocks the passage of sperms.

Q Is there any test for this?

A The postcoital test can be performed. Sexual intercourse is performed as close as possible to the release of the egg (between day 12 and day 16 of the menstrual cycle), when the mucus is clear and stringy. In the doctor's office later, a small amount of this mucus is then removed and examined under a microscope. There should be sperms swimming forwards through the mucus if all is well.

One problem with using clomiphene to treat poor egg release is that sometimes the amount of mucus produced by the cervix is reduced. This makes it difficult for sperms to pass through the cervix to enter the womb.

Problems with the tubes

Q   What causes disease of the tubes? How does this interfere with fertility?

A   Blockage of the Fallopian tubes can occur from previous infection of the reproductive organs (pelvic inflammatory disease) or from endometriosis. Imagine the Fallopian tube as a garden hose. An infection of the inside of the tube (endosalpingitis) can cause the inside to be choked or sealed off so that the egg cannot travel through it to meet the sperm. Sometimes, endometriosis or infection of the tissues outside the womb would cause the outer ends of the tubes near the ovaries to be gummed up or stuck to the intestines. This again prevents the egg from entering the tube.

Q   How do we know if the tubes are blocked?

A   This can be diagnosed through a special X-ray called a hysterosalpingogram (HSG). The patient lies down on an X-ray table while a dye is injected into the neck of the womb. The doctor then looks at an X-ray screen to see if the dye passes through the tubes.

Q   Is this painful?

A   This procedure is done without anaesthesia and is slightly uncomfortable. Here is a first-person account:

I lay in isolation on this cold table in the X-ray room, wondering where everybody else was. A collection of cold machines stood nearby. Was I the only human being in this room? I felt out-numbered. Soon, my gynaecologist came in, wearing what looked like an armour plate. He looked part machine, part human to me. That was half a consolation. As he explained the procedure to me, he was quite his human self and I felt better.

First, some cleaning solution was used to wipe the vagina. I felt a little discomfort as he used an instrument to hold the neck of my womb before injecting the dye.

We looked at a big TV screen and there the dye was, spreading up and coming through what my gynaecologist said were my tubes. As the dye passed out of the tubes, I felt a dull ache in my lower tummy, just like during my menses.

I got off the cold table, happy with the knowledge that my tubes were fine, and marvelling at what man and machine could do together. I bled a little for 2 days but other than that, I was fine.

Poor hormone secretion by the ovaries (luteal phase defects)

Q What is luteal phase defect?

A Commonly called 'weak ovaries', this condition occurs when the ovaries produce insufficient amounts of the hormone progesterone after the release of the egg. Progesterone is important, among other reasons, for causing the lining of the womb to produce glycogen. Glycogen nourishes the embryo after it enters the womb. Low levels of the hormone would then affect the attachment of the embryo to the womb.

Q   How can this be confirmed and treated?

A   You would remember that in a menstrual cycle where the woman produces an egg, her temperature rises for the duration of the second half of the cycle. When taking the basal body temperature, a poor rise in the second half of the menstrual cycle would indicate luteal phase defect. This can be confirmed by a blood test for progesterone on day 22 of the cycle and by taking a small sample of tissue from inside the womb for examination.

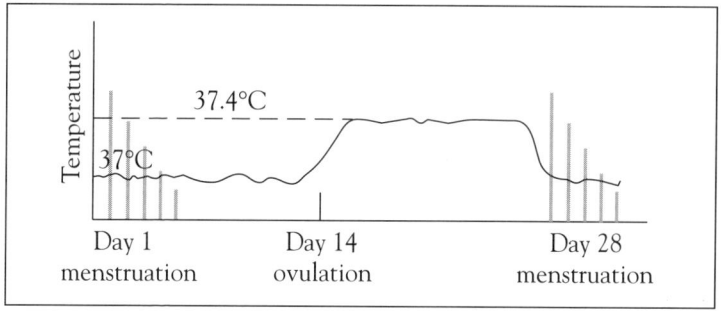

Note how body temperature changes in a menstrual cycle.

The good news is that luteal phase defect, unlike tubal disease, is usually a temporary condition in most women. If persistent, it can be treated either via tablets placed in the vagina (progesterone pessaries) or intramuscular injections given 3 days after the temperature rises. This treatment is repeated until the menstruation occurs or until pregnancy is confirmed.

Problems with the womb

Q   What conditions of the womb can prevent pregnancy?

A   Infections of the womb by the bacteria which causes
tuberculosis (TB) of the lungs or by a germ *called
T mycoplasma* can affect fertility. Abnormal wombs which are
present from birth are another reason. In these cases, there
may be two wombs and the inside lining so deformed that
attachment of the embryo is affected. Similarly, fibroids (non-
cancerous growths of the uterus) and polyps (growths
attached to the wall of the womb by a narrow stalk) can also
affect attachment of the embryo. If the fibroids are located
near the part where the Fallopian tube enters the womb then
they can cause blockage of the tube.

Q   How are these conditions treated?

A   Infections are treated with the appropriate antibiotics. For
abnormal wombs or growths inside the womb, an
operation is needed.

Q   What is a tilted womb?

A   This refers to a retroverted uterus, where the top of the
womb is displaced backwards instead of forwards.

Q   I have a tilted womb. Can I get pregnant?

A   A retroverted uterus does not usually affect fertility. It also
does not complicate delivery. However, you may
experience pain on deep penetration during intercourse.

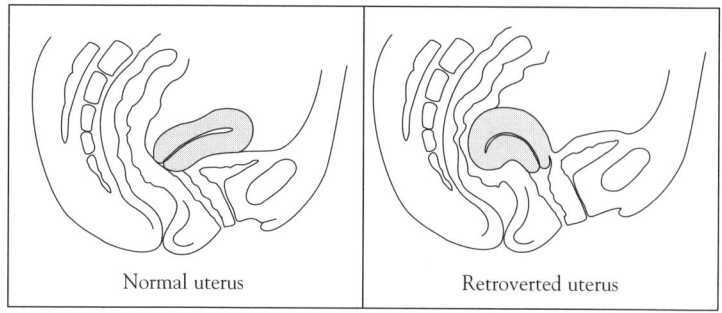

| Normal uterus | Retroverted uterus |

Normal and retroverted wombs

Causes of infertility in the male

Q Is male infertility a big problem?

A Data accumulated over the last 20 years reveal that in approximately 20 per cent of all couples evaluated for failure to conceive, a significant problem was found in the man alone. In another 20 per cent, an abnormality was present in both the man and the woman. Thus, in approximately 40 per cent of infertile couples, the man was at least partly responsible for the failure to conceive.

Q What are the causes of male infertility?

A These can be conveniently grouped into two categories, namely problems with sexual intercourse and problems with semen quality.

Q What are the common problems with sexual intercourse?

A These include a failure to maintain erection of the penis (impotence) and premature ejaculation. Occasionally, following an operation of the urinary passage in the man, semen flows backwards into the bladder during ejaculation instead of forwards out of the penis (retrograde ejaculation).

 What is a seminal analysis?

This is the examination of a sample of semen under a microscope. The following are normal values for a semen analysis.

Normal values for semen analysis

Volume of ejaculate	1.5 to 5 ml
Sperm density	more than 20 million/ml
Percentage of live sperms	more than 60%
Sperm movement	more than 50% moving forwards
Sperm appearance	more than 60% of normal looking sperms

No significant clumping together of sperms

No significant amount of pus cells in the semen

No significant amount of blood in the semen

 What are the precautions necessary for collecting a sample of semen?

Semen has to be properly collected for the analysis to be valid. All specimens should be collected after a period of abstinence of 2 to 3 days and taken to the laboratory within 2 hours. The specimen should be collected in a glass bottle following masturbation, or following sexual intercourse. In the latter case, the penis is withdrawn just prior to ejaculation and the ejaculate collected directly in a clean glass bottle.

Q What are the ways in which semen quality can be improved?

A It is important for a man who is trying to father a child to keep in good health as semen quality to some extent depends on the general health of the man. Viral infections with high fever affects sperm count and movement. Heat is damaging for sperms. The sitting position pushes the testes close to the body and body heat is detrimental to sperms. Occupations which involve long hours of sitting are not good for a man with poor sperm quality. Studies have shown that all else being equal, bus drivers have fewer children than bus conductors. Sauna baths and hot tubs are also out, just as tight briefs are. Boxer shorts are in as they are loose and therefore allow the testes to hang down where the temperature is lower. Other activities like smoking and excessive alcohol consumption are also bad for sperm quality.

Q Is it possible to have no sperms in the ejaculate?

A Azoospermia is the word used to describe an ejaculate which contains no sperms. In army terms, this is called firing blanks.

Q What causes azoospermia?

A There are three causes for azoospermia.
These are:

- Failure of the testes to produce sperms. This can be the result of failure of the testes to develop since birth or from infections like mumps in adulthood. In the former condition, the testes are very small on examination whereas in the latter situation, the testes can be of normal size.

- Obstruction along the genital tract. The passage along which sperms travel (the vas deferens) may be undeveloped or blocked since birth. This occurs in 10 per cent of azoospermic patients.

- Abnormal ejaculation where semen flows backwards into the bladder.

Understanding how it works

Q What is the role of the cervix in infertility?

A The cervix plays an important role in fertility. Mucus produced by cells in the cervix protects sperms from the hostile acidic environment of the vagina. The mucus also supplements the energy requirements of the sperms and provides the proper environment for the sperms to penetrate and fertilize the egg. Perhaps the most important function of the cervix is as a sperm reservoir. Only occasionally does coitus occur at ovulation. The cervix then stores the sperms and allows a steady release so that there is a constant supply of sperms at the site of fertilization for many hours before and after ovulation.

Q What is the postcoital test?

A This is a test which is done as closely as possible to the time of ovulation as determined by the body temperature and changes in the cervical mucus. The couple is instructed to refrain from intercourse for 2 days prior to the test, which is performed 6 to 10 hours after the sexual intercourse.

With the patient lying down on the examination couch, a speculum is inserted into the vagina and a sample of vaginal fluid taken and examined for sperms. The reason for examining the vaginal fluid is to check that sperms are actually deposited in the vagina after intercourse. (Unfortunately, not everybody has the same idea of what intercourse should be!)

Using a different syringe, some mucus is taken from inside the cervix. This mucus is placed under a separate glass slide and examined under a microscope. In a normal test, live sperms should be seen swimming purposefully through the cervical mucus.

When nature needs a helping hand

Q What is artificial insemination?

A Artificial insemination is the process of fertilization apart from normal sexual intercourse. There are two forms of artificial insemination. One is artificial insemination by the husband (AIH), whereby sperms from the husband are placed in the patient's vagina during the period of ovulation to allow spontaneous conception. The other is artificial insemination by a donor, when sperms from another man is used for fertilization. The former method is used when the husband has a normal semen analysis but is unable to deposit sperms naturally either because of impotence or retrograde ejaculation. The latter method is used when the husband has azoospermia, making it necessary to obtain semen from someone other than the husband.

Q What is GIFT?

A Gamete IntraFallopian Transfer or GIFT is a form of assisted conception for couples having difficulty in conceiving spontaneously. The patient is first made to produce many eggs in her ovary by the use of drugs. At the time when these eggs are about to be released, she is brought into the operating theatre for the procedure.

The patient is anaesthetized and 10 to 12 eggs sucked out from her ovaries using a very fine needle attached to an ultrasound machine. The best egg is then chosen and mixed with the husband's semen which had been prepared 2 hours earlier so that only active sperms are used. The egg-and-sperm mixture is then carefully injected into the outer portion of the Fallopian tube using a laparoscope. The whole procedure takes about 45 minutes and the patient is able to go home the same day.

Q What is IVF?

A In-Vitro Fertilization or IVF is another assisted reproductive technique. It is different from GIFT in that fertilization occurs outside the body. In this procedure, the patient is again prepared by stimulation of the ovaries with drugs so that many follicles are produced. The patient is then sedated and the eggs extracted through the vagina. The eggs are then mixed with prepared sperms and fertilization occurs in a little glass container. Two days later, the embryo is injected into the womb of the woman and she can then go home the same day. Progesterone is given for the next 2 weeks to help in implantation of the embryo.

Q What are the success rates of these procedures?

A The success rates of GIFT and IVF vary from centre to centre and an average value would be a 30 per cent pregnancy rate per cycle. However, miscarriages may occur so that the chances of bringing a baby home is actually lower.

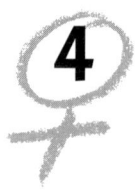

4

Losing a Pre-term Baby

'I'm 8 weeks pregnant and bleeding heavily. What should I do?'
There is nothing more frightening for a newly pregnant woman
than the sight of blood on a panty liner. The terrifying fear of a
miscarriage rears its ugly head and the joy of pregnancy quickly
vanishes.

Q What is a miscarriage?

A A miscarriage is the loss of the baby before 28 weeks of
pregnancy. The medical term is spontaneous abortion,
which can be divided into two groups: early or first trimester
(those occurring within the first 12 weeks of pregnancy) and
late or second trimester (those occurring between 12 and
28 weeks pregnancy).

Q What are the signs of an impending miscarriage?

A Bleeding is the most significant danger signal that all is
not right with a pregnancy. This may begin first as a
brownish stain which quickly turns to red. Pain, especially a
low cramp, is a bad sign if it accompanies an increased
amount of bleeding as this may signal the start of a
miscarriage.

Early miscarriages

Q What can cause an early miscarriage?

A An abnormal fetus is the commonest cause of an early miscarriage. Other reasons include infections by viruses, diseases like diabetes, 'weak' ovaries (see luteal phase defects) and an abnormal womb. However, in many instances, no actual cause for the miscarriage can be found. Excessive physical or mental stress in early pregnancy has been associated with an increased risk of early miscarriages. This is why it is not advisable to work too hard during the first 12 weeks of pregnancy.

Q What kind of infection can cause a miscarriage?

A Infections which are caused by viruses have been linked to miscarriages. In particular, that which causes German measles (rubella), herpes (a kind of sexually transmitted disease) and another called the cytomegalovirus (CMV), have been associated with early pregnancy losses. Infection by a parasite called *Toxoplasma*, which is associated with cats, has also been known to cause miscarriages.

Q What is the treatment for bleeding in early pregnancy?

A An ultrasound examination is first conducted to make sure that there is a gestational sac inside the womb. Strict bed rest, preferably in hospital, is then advised. Regular injections with a hormone called human chorionic gonadotrophin (HCG) would decrease the chances of a miscarriage if the cause of the bleeding is 'weak' ovaries. If the fetus is normal and there is nothing wrong with the womb, then the bleeding would gradually decrease to a brown stain and eventually stop. Regular tests to measure the level of the pregnancy hormone, beta HCG, in the blood is also done. Increasing levels indicate that the pregnancy is progressing normally. Symptoms of early pregnancy like nausea and vomiting may then increase and the patient can be discharged from hospital. She is given medical leave to rest at home for a further period to allow the pregnancy to stabilize.

Q What if the bleeding increases despite treatment?

A Increased bleeding with accompanying low abdominal cramps is a bad sign. If this is accompanied by falling levels of the pregnancy hormone beta HCG, then a vaginal examination is done. If the neck of the womb begins to open, then a miscarriage is about to occur. The medical term for this is inevitable abortion.

Q What does a miscarriage actually feel like?

A Usually, the low abdominal pain increases in intensity to become strong rhythmic cramps, accompanied by the 'urge to pass motion'. The patient may feel nauseous or even vomit, and a small piece of fleshy tissue (like raw liver) is passed out of the vagina. The low abdominal pain and nausea immediately stops and the bleeding decreases.

Q What needs to be done after a miscarriage?

A After the fetus has been passed out, the womb has to be cleaned out to prevent infection as small parts of the pregnancy may still be left inside. A minor operation called a dilatation and curettage (D & C) needs to be done.

The patient is given a general anaesthesia and the opening of the womb (cervix) dilated with a metal instrument to allow the entry of a plastic sucker tube. The remnant material inside the womb is sucked out. The inside of the womb is then scraped clean with another metal instrument called a curette, which looks like a small spoon.

 Is the procedure painful?

The patient feels no pain as the whole process is done under anaesthesia. Here is a first-person account of a patient who went through a D & C:

I was 7 weeks pregnant when I passed out the baby. I was numb with grief when they placed me on the table. A mask was put over my face and as I breathed in, I smelled something slightly sweet. I saw some flickering lights and then everything went black.

The next minute, someone was slapping my face and telling me to wake up. I was then pushed out of the operating theatre to the ward where my husband was waiting for me. My lower abdomen and vagina felt slightly sore and there was fresh blood on the sanitary towel. I still felt groggy and slept through the night.

The next day, I felt much better. My appetite had returned and the pain in my lower tummy was almost gone. I felt a little pain on passing urine. My gynaecologist then examined me and told me that my womb had almost returned to its normal size. The bleeding was much reduced and I was then allowed to go home.

 Are there any immediate complications after a D & C?

Infection of the womb can sometimes occur. The warning signs are low abdominal pain, increased bleeding or foul-smelling vaginal discharge and fever. This condition should be quickly treated otherwise blockage of the Fallopian tubes may occur later, with resultant infertility.

Q How long does it take for the bleeding to stop?

A The vaginal bleeding after a D & C usually lasts for one week. After the procedure, the bleeding gets less and turns from red to brown. Any increase in bleeding later is not normal. After the bleeding stops, the next menstruation would return between 4 and 6 weeks after the day of the D & C.

Q Is this the same D & C done for a woman who does not want a baby?

A For a wilful abortion, the procedure is essentially the same except that the process is done more forcefully. Hence complications, especially in later years, are more likely to occur. In such cases, infection, kidney damage and even death from anaesthesia have been known to occur during the actual operation. As the neck of the womb needs to be forcibly opened in patients who do not want the baby, damage to the neck of the womb (cervix) can happen. This leads to a 'weak womb', with a much higher chance of miscarriages in later pregnancies. As the scraping is also done more vigorously, the wall of the womb may be damaged, with the risk of rupture of the womb when the woman becomes pregnant again or during the next labour. Infection of the tubes may happen, leading to infertility.

For these and other reasons, wilful abortions are not advisable. Many times, a couple reason that they are 'not ready' yet for the baby as the flat or car has not been paid for. It is not difficult to keep the baby and make the necessary adjustments in life-style. This is because a wilful abortion is not something to be taken lightly. Apart from snuffing out an innocent life, there is the possibility of serious complications.

Also, it is not uncommon that after the 5 Cs have been attained, the baby just will not come. Now THAT is a real tragedy.

Q What is the purpose of doing an ultrasound scan when there is bleeding in early pregnancy?

A It is important to check that the pregnancy is inside the womb. Sometimes, the pregnancy settles outside the womb in the Fallopian tube (ectopic pregnancy). This is a grave medical emergency as the patient may die from internal bleeding.

Q What are the signs of an ectopic pregnancy?

A The patient usually complains of vaginal bleeding with low abdominal pain. In more serious cases, there would be difficulty in breathing, dizziness, fainting, nausea and cold sweats. An internal examination by the doctor would cause great pain when the neck of the womb is moved.

Q What needs to be done in such an instance?

A The patient needs to be sent immediately to a hospital which is equipped for an immediate operation. Here is a first-person account:

My period was 2 weeks overdue so I carried out a pregnancy test with a kit I had bought from a pharmacy. It was positive! I was elated.

The very next day, I noticed some dark red blood on my underwear. I decided to rest at home. That same afternoon, I had this horrific sharp sudden pain on the left side of my tummy. It got much worse and I could hardly walk. I called my gynaecologist, who asked me to rush down immediately to the clinic.

After examining me, he performed an ultrasound scan. He was frowning and told me that he could not see the pregnancy inside the womb. Instead, he saw a collection of fluid outside the womb which could mean that I was bleeding internally. He immediately called his nurse to alert the operating theatre and to call for the anaesthetist. In the meantime, he explained to me that there was a high probability that the pregnancy was in the left Fallopian tube and that an immediate operation with the laparoscope was necessary.

As my husband frantically called my office to inform them that I would be off work for a few days, my gynaecologist inserted a drip into a vein on my left hand. I was then wheeled from the clinic to the hospital. At that time, I began to feel dizzy and found it was getting difficult to breathe. My husband, who was accompanying me, noticed that I was very pale. The next I knew, there was this operating room and people in green were running around. The anaesthetist placed a mask over my face and I felt a warm gush in the vein of my left hand. Then I blacked out.

When I awoke, I was back in the hospital room and felt sore over my tummy. My husband said that there were three plasters over my tummy. My gynaecologist then appeared and told me that I was very fortunate. The pregnancy had burst through the left Fallopian tube and caused internal bleeding. There had been about four cupfuls of blood which had to be removed. He had located the pregnancy and removed it through the laparoscope to stop the bleeding but I still had my left Fallopian tube.

The next day, I felt slightly sore over the tummy but was able to eat. A nurse took some blood for examination. Later, I was told that my haemoglobin level was 9. I did not feel dizzy any more and was allowed to go home in the evening.

Q   I have had three early miscarriages. What should I do?

A   Recurrent early miscarriages usually occur when the fetus is not normal in each pregnancy. The chance of this happening is usually random in each instance. The usual causes of an early miscarriage such as infections or diseases like diabetes should be looked for and treated. An X-ray test called a hysterosalpingogram (HSG) is done to exclude an abnormal womb. Blood tests for abnormal chromosomes (the structure on which our genes are carried) should be done for both your husband and yourself. This is important because even though you are both normal, you could be carriers of an abnormal amount of genes.

Having done all the necessary tests, it is common to come up against a blank wall – the doctor can find no cause for the miscarriage. If such is the case, take heart and be optimistic for the next pregnancy. After one miscarriage, the chance of a second miscarriage is 12 per cent. After two miscarriages, the chance of another miscarriage rises to 16 per cent and after a third miscarriage the chance of a similar occurrence is 21 per cent. To put it differently, the chance of a miscarriage NOT occurring is then 79 per cent.

However, once another pregnancy is diagnosed, then additional precautionary steps are necessary. This includes bed rest, avoidance of alcohol and smoking, keeping away from people who are unwell with infectious diseases and regular injections of the hormone HCG. This has been shown to decrease the risk of subsequent miscarriages.

Late miscarriages

Q What can cause a late miscarriage?

A This occurs between 12 and 28 weeks of pregnancy. The causes are somewhat different from that of an early miscarriage. The causes include weakness of the neck of the womb (the cervix) as well as abnormal shape of the womb which has been present from birth. This makes it difficult for the womb to contain the fetus and grow with the pregnancy, hence causing a late miscarriage.

Q What can cause weakness of the neck of the womb?

A This is usually due to previous operations on the neck of the womb. In particular, a previous wilful abortion where the neck of the womb had to be forcibly opened to more than one centimeter may permanently damage the cervix. Sometimes, a woman may have had an operation called a cone biopsy for precancerous disease of the neck of the womb. This can also lead to damage and late miscarriages.

Q How can we treat this condition?

A At 13 weeks of pregnancy, a minor operation is performed. The patient is put under general anaesthesia and a stitch of elastic tape is placed into the neck of the womb to keep it closed. The patient is then hospitalized for a few days. This stitch is then removed at 38 weeks of pregnancy so that a normal delivery is possible.

What about abnormal wombs?

 These are usually abnormalities which are present from birth (congenital abnormalities) and include a double womb or a womb with a partition in the inside. This makes it difficult for the fetus to grow and enlarge within it, and hence late miscarriages may occur.

What is the treatment for an abnormal womb?

This involves a more major operation in which the abnormal partition is removed and the edges of the womb stitched together. This gives one internal space which is larger than the two smaller spaces previously.

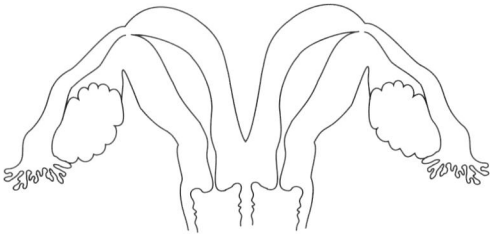

Double uterus, cervix and vagina

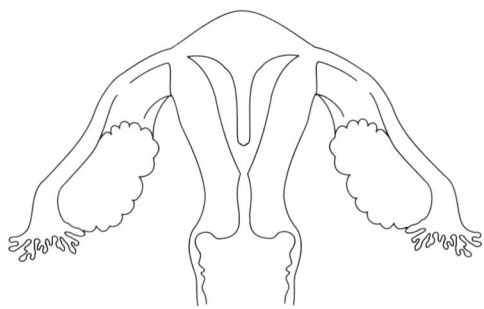

Uterus with a partition inside

Q What are the signs of a late miscarriage?

A The patient usually complains of sticky bleeding from the vagina or the passing of a large amount of clear fluid which is not urine. Pain is usually not as severe as in early miscarriages. If it does happen, it is rhythmic and cramp-like, rather like labour pain. The whole baby is then passed out and the afterbirth (the placenta) follows soon after.

Q What needs to be done after a late miscarriage?

A The same procedure of cleaning the womb as in an early miscarriage, i.e. a D & C, needs to be done as parts of the placenta are likely to be left behind.

Q My friend said she had a miscarriage where she passed out some 'grapes'. What is that?

A She appears to have had a molar pregnancy. This is a condition where there is no fetus but instead excessive growth of the placental tissues. Apart from the fact that no healthy baby will arise from this conception, there is a chance of a cancer developing.

Q What needs to be done?

A The pregnancy must be terminated quickly with a D & C. Thereafter, regular blood tests are done to measure the pregnancy hormone HCG. After the D & C, the levels of this hormone should reach zero within 12 weeks. Failure to do so indicates that a cancer called choriocarcinoma has developed. Once the hormone has reached zero, your friend should be told to avoid pregnancy for at least a year as the cancer may develop later.

After a miscarriage ...

Q What foods should be taken after a miscarriage?

A A diet rich in protein and iron should be taken to enable the body to replenish the blood lost in the miscarriage. Chinese herbs in a tonic soup which is tasty may stimulate a poor appetite. On the following page are recipes which provide high-grade protein. These recipes could serve equally well for the post-delivery period.

Q How does one get over the grief of a miscarriage?

A A miscarriage is an extremely painful physical, emotional and psychological experience as it involves the death of what would have otherwise been a close member of the family. Face the situation squarely, with the comfort that the child was in all likelihood abnormal to start with. Tears are a natural response and the more the better. Bottling up and suppressing grief delays one's recovery and resumption of a normal life. Life goes on, the pain subsides and before long, a missed period would herald another pregnancy.

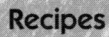

Recipes

Double-boiled beef soup

You need:
¹/₂ kg of shin beef cut into ³/₄-inch cubes
4 or 5 cups of water

1. Put the beef cubes and water into a double boiler. Add salt to taste.
2. Let it boil for 3 to 4 hours.

Eight-treasure soup

You need:
a spring chicken cut into halves or quarters
babao, which is made of 8 types of herbs: *hongzao*, *huaishan*, *baihe*, *qizi*, *yuzhu*, *dangshen*, *longyan* and *chuanxiong*; *babao* is available at Chinese medical shops at about $2.50 per packet
4 or 5 cups of water

1. Put the chicken, herbs and water into a double boiler. Add a little salt to bring out the flavour.
2. Let it boil for 3 to 4 hours.

5 Expecting a Baby

'Darling, I feel a little nauseous this morning.'
'Don't worry. Must be the oysters you had last night.'
'I've also missed my period.'
Klunk! He faints.

This is an extremely exciting time for the couple – a missed period, nausea and a positive urine pregnancy test.

The first three months

Q How soon can a pregnancy be diagnosed?

A A pregnancy can be diagnosed even before a missed period. With a blood test, it can be diagnosed on day 21 of the cycle. With the usual urine pregnancy test, a positive diagnosis can be made a few days after the expected period is due. However, it is important to use an early morning specimen of urine.

Q What are the earliest symptoms of pregnancy?

A The first symptoms usually appear at 5 weeks from the first day of the last menstruation. These include a funny taste in the mouth and a change in appetite. This is usually accompanied by a tingling sensation of the nipples as the breasts become more sensitive. Nausea and vomiting is a common experience in most patients and begins at 6 to 7 weeks of pregnancy.

Q What is 'morning sickness'? How long does it last?

A Nausea and vomiting in early pregnancy is commonly called 'morning sickness'. This may not be an accurate description as many patients actually experience it in the evening while others vomit throughout the day! This condition often improves after 16 weeks of pregnancy.

Q Is morning sickness harmful for the patient?

A It is usually not, but if severe, can lead to dehydration. In such instances, the patient is hospitalized and a drip is set up to replace lost fluids.

Q If there is excessive vomiting, won't the fetus be deprived of nutrition?

A The fetus is usually spared any ill effects because whatever it needs in the form of nutrition is obtained from stores in the mother. That is why vitamin supplements, especially folic acid, is given to a pregnant woman.

Q What causes morning sickness?

A The hormones of pregnancy released by the developing placenta slows down the muscles of the organs of the digestive system like the stomach and intestines. This is believed to be a main cause of nausea and vomiting. It also often causes constipation in pregnancy.

Q What should a woman do when she has morning sickness?

A She should eat small quantities of food at more frequent intervals. Instead of three large meals a day, six smaller meals would be more appropriate. She should also eat what tickles her fancy as practically all foods would have some nutritional value.

Q What foods should she avoid?

A She should avoid foodstuffs which are too oily, like fried kuay teow or fried oyster omelette, as oily foods would hinder digestion. Spicy and chillied food should also be taken in moderation as it makes vomiting acutely unpleasant. Raw food or meals which have been prepared in unhygienic conditions should also be avoided as the last thing we want is for a pregnant woman to come down with food poisoning and diarrhoea.

Q What medication can be used for morning sickness?

A There are many types of medicines for treating morning sickness. These are actually similar to those used for motion or travel sickness. They are in tablet form and safe for the developing fetus. For more severe vomiting where little or no food can be retained if swallowed, the patient is placed on an intravenous drip and the medication given through the drip.

Vitamin B complex tablets or injections can also reduce nausea and vomiting.

Q My friend had blood in her vomit. Is this serious?

A This is quite common, especially after she has vomited several times. In the course of vomiting, the muscles above the stomach contract and this leads to blood vessels bursting. Although frightening, this condition is usually quite harmless and stops on its own.

However, if large amounts of blood is thrown up, then it indicates a more serious problem like a stomach ulcer. Medical attention is then needed.

Q What is heartburn?

A Heartburn is another common complaint in early pregnancy. It is caused by the relaxation of the muscular valve just above the stomach as a result of pregnancy hormones. The patient feels a burning sensation which is typically worse when she lies down because the acid from the stomach then flows upwards. This is treated with antacids which are either in tablet or liquid form. Regular meals also dilute the acid and make heartburn less severe.

Q I feel like there is a lot of gas in my tummy. Why is this so?

A The hormones of pregnancy cause the muscles of the stomach and intestines to slow down. A lot of swallowed air gets trapped instead of being passed through the intestines and hence, the general feeling of bloatedness. This usually eases after the first 14 weeks.

Q Is vaginal discharge common in early pregnancy?

A It is normal to have increased vaginal discharge in pregnancy. This is usually white or slightly yellow. Discharge that is thick like yoghurt, green or accompanied by an itch is not normal and may indicate a yeast infection.

Q I am 10 weeks pregnant and experiencing cramps in the lower tummy. Why is this so?

A Lower abdominal pain or discomfort is common in early pregnancy and is caused by the womb enlarging. When this happens, the blood vessels around the womb also swell and stimulation of the nerves around them causes the pain. There are also two ligaments like thick rubber bands which stretch from the front of the womb to the front of the lower abdomen. These are called the round ligaments. The stretching of these ligaments as the womb enlarges also contribute to the pain. Sometimes, a pain in the lower abdomen can be caused by infection of the bladder.

Q Is pain the only feeling when there is infection of the bladder?

A Infection of the bladder (cystitis) is more common in pregnancy. Usually there is pain over the lower abdomen, associated with the feeling of always wanting to go to the toilet. Each time, however, only a small amount of urine is passed and the passage of urine is accompanied by a burning sensation. Sometimes, the urine is cloudy or may be pinkish red from blood. Fever is present in more serious cases and if accompanied by chills or shivering, then the infection is more serious and may involve the kidneys.

Q How can this condition be treated?

A First, a urine sample is collected and sent to the laboratory to identify the bacteria so that the correct antibiotic can be given. Antibiotics of the penicillin group are usually effective for this condition and are safe for the baby. In more serious cases where there is infection of the kidneys, the antibiotic may need to be given through a drip.

Q When is it necessary to be hospitalized for low abdominal pain?

A Low abdominal pain is common in pregnancy and is usually not serious, especially if it comes once in a long while. However, hospitalization may be necessary if pain is accompanied by bleeding as it may indicate a pregnancy in the Fallopian tube or a possibility of miscarriage. Pain which is continuous or which gets worse may be caused by appendicitis. This makes it necessary for the patient to be hospitalized.

Q Is it safe to have sex in early pregnancy?

A In the absence of bleeding in early pregnancy, it is generally safe to have sexual intercourse. However, it is best to refrain until after the 12th week because of the possibility of infection. During intercourse, germs from around the anus can be pushed close to the neck of the womb. Also, the excessive physical movement may not be good for the developing fetus. Lastly, semen contains hormones which, together with the female orgasm, cause mild contractions of the womb. If necessary, it is advisable to have a good wash before intercourse and to use the condom.

Q What about air travel in early pregnancy?

A This is generally safe in the absence of bleeding. However, when flying above the clouds, there is more radiation from the sun and this is theoretically not good for the developing fetus. Also, air pockets may cause severe bumping. It is advisable to avoid all trips until after the 12th week. If it is necessary to travel, keep the trips short. Long journeys only add to the fatigue usually present during the early days of pregnancy.

Q Can I play tennis in early pregnancy?

A Strenuous activities which involve running or jumping should be avoided in early pregnancy. The body requires energy for the growing fetus. Also, the fetus is attached to the wall of the womb by the umbilical cord which is only as thick as a strand of *mianxian* (wheat vermicelli). Any excessive movement is theoretically bad. If you need to play golf, practise the chip and putt for 9 months; no 300 yard drives. Your handicap would probably be lowered after the delivery!

Q What is the use of an ultrasound scan in early pregnancy?

A An ultrasound scan is done to locate the pregnancy sac in the womb. This will exclude a pregnancy in the Fallopian tube which can sometimes occur with no pain or vaginal bleeding. Also, the size of the fetus can be accurately determined and from this, the expected date of delivery can be worked out. This is especially important in a patient with irregular menstruation.

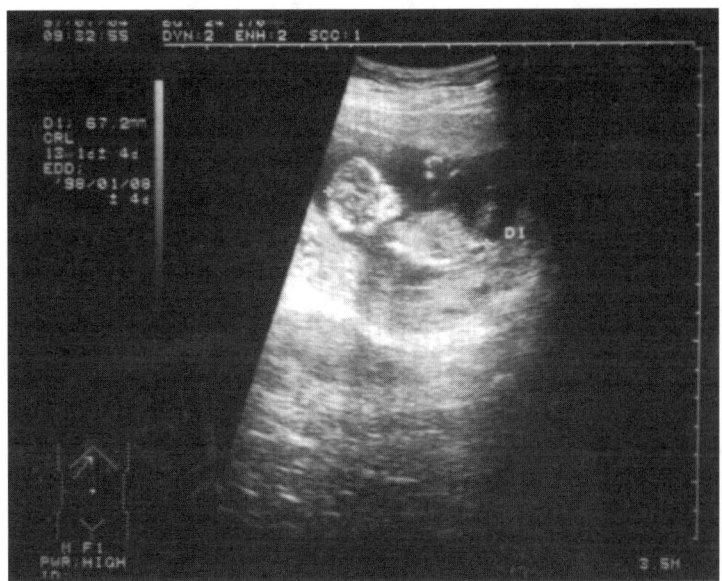

This is one for baby's photo album – an ultrasound scan of a fetus at 13 weeks. You can make out the head and body of the fetus fairly easily.

Q Is an ultrasound scan safe in early pregnancy?

A This is safe as sound waves similar to those used in dog whistles and not strong X-rays are used. When comparing babies who were exposed to ultrasound scans in the womb and those who were not, there was no difference in the number of abnormal babies in the two groups.

Q What blood tests are done in early pregnancy?

A Routine blood tests include the full blood count and thalassaemia screening, rubella IgG, VDRL, hepatitis B antigen and antibody, fasting blood sugar, ABO and Rhesus blood group, hepatitis C virus and anti-HIV. The full blood count is done to detect anaemia and Rubella IgG to determine immunity to German measles. The VDRL is for the diagnosis of latent syphilis which would lead to abnormalities in the baby if not treated. The blood sugar test is done to exclude diabetes. Hepatitis C is a relatively new disease which can cause progressive damage to the liver. The anti-HIV test is to detect AIDS as the baby needs special care if the virus is present in the mother.

Q What can be done to detect abnormal babies in early pregnancy?

A A complicated test called chorionic villus sampling (CVS)is done at 10 to 11 weeks to detect abnormalities like Down's syndrome. In this test, the patient is placed on a table and a thin metal tube inserted through the vagina into the neck of the womb. Using gentle suction, some material from the pregnancy is extracted and placed into a glass dish. This is then sent to the laboratory for examination. The advantage of this test is that serious abnormalities of the baby can be detected early, but the disadvantage is that there is a danger of miscarriage. This risk varies from 2 to 10 per cent, depending on the skill of the doctor.

From the fourth month onwards

With the discomforts of the first 3 months behind her, the pregnant woman begins to really enjoy her pregnancy. She eats well, looks radiant and her eyes sparkle. It's like being in love all over again. This is especially so for the second trimester (from 12 weeks to 28 weeks) as the womb is not too large to cause much discomfort and she is still able to pass through the supermarket turnstiles without too much difficulty.

Q Is it safe to drive in pregnancy?

A It is safe to do so but please drive slowly and carefully. The reflexes of a pregnant woman are slower and she therefore needs more time to react to traffic situations.

Also, please always wear a seat belt. The fetus may suffer damage if the uterus hits the steering wheel during an accident.

Q Is there any test to screen for an abnormal fetus?

A The triple test is used as a screening test for Down's syndrome (mongolism) and other similar abnormalities. This blood test is performed between 15 and 18 weeks of pregnancy and measures the level of three hormones in the blood of the pregnant woman. Hence the name triple test. The odds of the patient carrying a baby with mongolism are then calculated through a computer. A positive test means the risk is greater than 1 in 250. It must be stressed that this is useful as a screening test but is not always accurate, i.e. it may give a positive result in a woman with a perfectly normal baby.

Q What needs to be done in such a case?

A When a triple test gives a positive result or when the pregnant woman is more than 35 years old, then a more accurate test called amniocentesis is done. This is carried out between 16 and 18 weeks of pregnancy. The patient lies horizontally on the examination couch and the skin of the abdomen wiped with iodine to kill the surface germs. An ultrasound scanner is then used to determine the position of the placenta and the fetus. A local anaesthetic is then injected into the skin. Next, a long needle is introduced into the water bag, avoiding the fetus and placenta. Amniotic fluid is then withdrawn from the water bag and the needle removed. A plaster is placed over the skin and the fluid is sent to the laboratory.

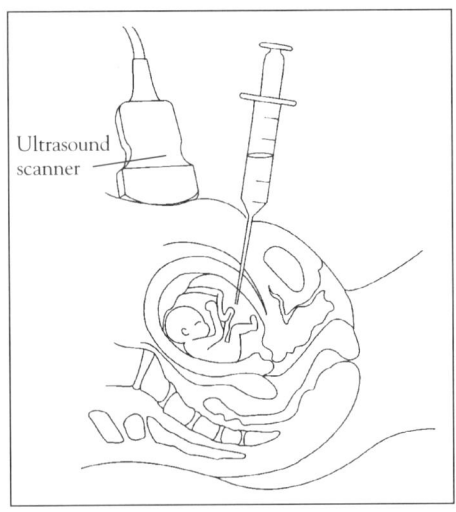

In amniocentesis, the ultrasound scanner is used to check the position of the placenta and fetus so that the needle does not touch the fetus.

 Is there any risk in amniocentesis?

As in all medical procedures, a small risk is involved. The complication rate varies from 0.5 to 2 per cent. This includes leakage of the water bag, infection and early labour, with loss of the fetus. Hence, amniocentesis is only advised when the risk of Down's syndrome is greater than the risk of the procedure.

Here is a first-person account of a patient undergoing amniocentesis:

I was 40 years old and pregnant for the first time. My gynaecologist said that my risk of having a mongoloid child was 1 in 40. After much discussion with my husband, we decided to go ahead with the test and all its risks as we could not bear the thought of having an abnormal child.

I was very nervous, lying on the couch next to the ultrasound machine. My gynaecologist then cleaned my tummy with this cold brown liquid and put this white object, which he called the ultrasound scanner, on my tummy. We could see the baby swimming around. I subconsciously called out to my baby to get out of the way and give the doctor room to remove the fluid. I then felt a needle prick on my tummy as my gynaecologist gave me a pain-killing injection.

The room was curiously quiet as he said he was about to begin. I felt a sickening cold feeling as the needle was inserted. There was no pain but I felt a little nauseous. I then saw this light yellow liquid being sucked into a syringe and the whole process was over in less than a minute. My gynaecologist then wiped my tummy and put a plaster over the injection.

He then used another machine and I heard my baby's heart pumping. I even saw it on the scanner. Was I relieved! I was told to observe for pains in the tummy, fever or leaking of water through my vagina at home but thankfully, nothing happened. The 2-week wait for the results was sheer agony! Then one morning, I received a call from the clinic to say that the baby was a normal male. I wept with relief.

What is the purpose of an ultrasound scan in mid pregnancy?

This is done for three main reasons, namely to find the position of the placenta, to look for structural abnormalities of the fetus and to determine whether the fetus is growing normally through repeated scans.

Q What are the structural abnormalities which can be picked up with an ultrasound scan?

A Numerous abnormalities can be picked up with the ultrasound scan and these include hole in the heart, cleft lips, excessive fluid in the brain, abnormal brain structures, abnormal stomach or kidneys and short limbs. However, it must be stressed that only specialized centres with very sensitive machines will be able to detect small abnormalities.

Q How can the ultrasound machine show that the fetus is growing well?

A Repeated scans at 2-weekly intervals are done to determine whether the baby is growing well. The size of the head, waistline of the fetus and length of the long leg bone should increase in proportion. When the placenta gives the baby insufficient nutrition, the baby's waist would grow less in comparison with the head. The ratio of head size to waist size would increase and the doctor will be warned that closer monitoring of the baby would be necessary. Also, the level of fluid in the womb would decrease, which is another warning sign.

Q What are Braxton–Hicks contractions?

A Braxton–Hicks contractions are painless, irregular contractions of the womb which become more common after 30 weeks of pregnancy. They are different from true labour pains as they do not cause the neck of the womb to open up.

Q How can we treat these contractions?

A Bed rest and a drug called salbutamol is used to treat Braxton–Hicks contractions. The side-effect of salbutamol is heart palpitations.

Q I am 34 weeks pregnant and was told that I have a low-lying placenta. What does this mean?

A The placenta is the organ that connects the fetus to the mother. It is attached to the inner wall of the womb and serves to pass nutrients from mother to fetus and waste products from fetus to mother. In a low-lying placenta, (placenta previa), the position of the placenta is over the lower part of the womb, covering the neck of the womb. This can cause painless bleeding in the later part of pregnancy and may prevent normal delivery, in which case a Caesarean section is needed.

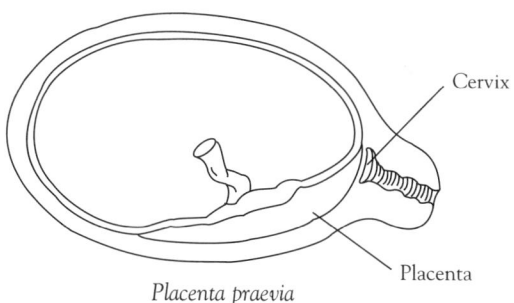

Cervix

Placenta

Placenta praevia

Q Is there any other cause for bleeding in later pregnancy?

A Another cause for bleeding in later pregnancy is a condition called abruptio placentae. In this instance, the placenta is detached from the inner wall of the womb by a large blood clot. The patient experiences bleeding, accom-panied by severe abdominal pain. There may also be absence of movement of the fetus. This condition is serious as the baby may die in the womb and the mother may bleed profusely because of failure of her blood to clot.

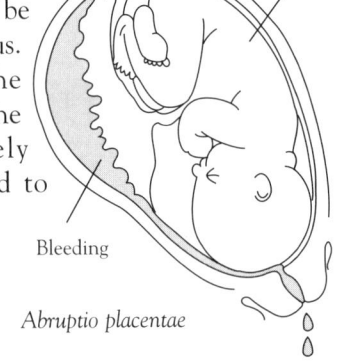

Abruptio placentae

Q Is backache common in later pregnancy?

A Aches and pains of the lower body are more common in later pregnancy. This is because the hormones of pregnancy which are secreted by the placenta causes a relaxation of all the ligaments in the body. Ligaments are like rubber bands which hold joints together. The loosening of these supporting bands mean that the joints are less well supported, therefore causing pain especially with movement. The main joints affected are those of the lower back and hip and the pain is usually worse when standing. It is relieved when the patient lies down. Central back pain is also made worse in later pregnancy when the weight of the enlarging womb causes the spine to curve forwards more. This imposes a strain on the nerves and joints of the lower back. Another joint which tends to hurt in later pregnancy is that of the pubic bone, just above where the patient passes urine. This is caused by stretching of the pubic joint as the fetal head enters the birth canal. Pain may be severe enough to prevent the patient from walking.

Q How can these pains be treated?

A The patient should rest more and avoid activities such as excessive walking, which aggravate the pain. If severe, paracetamol is safe and can be taken 3 times a day. Pain-relieving ointments or applications can also be used. Some patients find a hot water bottle helpful and this is laid over the painful joint.

Q I am 36 weeks pregnant and find it difficult to breathe when lying down. Why is this so?

A At 36 weeks, the top of the womb is just below the level of the rib cage. This prevents the lungs from expanding freely and hence gives rise to the feeling of breathlessness. If necessary, sleep on two or even three pillows.

Q I find it difficult to lie flat. Is there a need to do so?

A On the contrary, it is better to lie with the body at a slight tilt, either to the left or right side. This prevents the weight of the large womb from pressing on the big blood vessels running from the lower body to the heart. Pressure on these structures would cause dizzy spells as the amount of blood returning to the brain would be decreased. Also, blood supply to the placenta and hence the fetus may be reduced when the patient lies flat on her back.

Q What is a breech baby?

A In a breech presentation, the fetus lies in the womb with its head on top and the buttocks (or breech) below. At 32 weeks of pregnancy, 25 per cent of fetuses are lying in the breech presentation but at birth, only 4 per cent are so. This means that between 32 and 40 weeks, a large number of fetuses turn on their own to the head-down position.

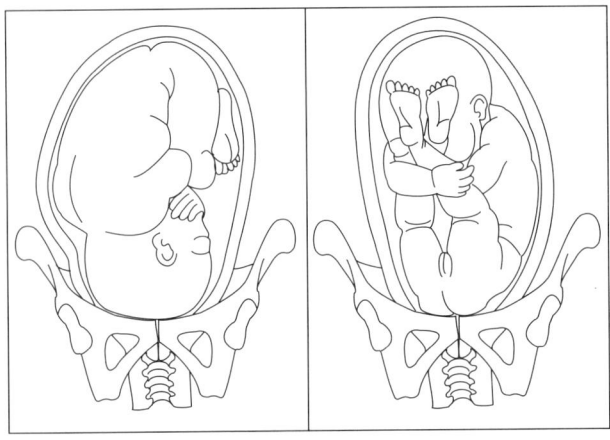

Left –
*normal
presentation*

Right –
*one of the
many forms
of breech
presentation*

 Is there any danger to a breech baby?

 The danger in a breech presentation occurs mainly at the time of delivery. The complications are mainly to the baby and include brain damage, dislocation of the neck, damage to the organs like the liver in the abdomen, fracture of the arms and legs, and dislocation of the hip and elbow joints. These complications are more likely in first-time deliveries or when the baby is large compared to the size of the mother. All said, a breech baby faces 10 times as much danger as a baby in a normal head-first delivery.

 How then should a breech baby be delivered?

Normal delivery through the vagina is still possible but great care must be taken before the onset of labour, to ensure that the baby is not too large as compared to the size of the pelvic bones of the mother. This includes ultrasound scanning of the baby's size and X-ray measurements of the pelvic bones. If the fetus is considered too large, then a Caesarean section would be necessary.

I remember the day when a tourist was carried into the emergency room in labour. She was 36 weeks pregnant. She said she felt something in the vagina and when she undressed, the nurse screamed! Two tiny feet were sticking out from her vagina! The baby was in a breech position and we quickly placed her on the couch and managed to deliver the baby. Just last week, she sent us a lovely card. The baby was one year old and she was 6 weeks pregnant again.

Q What is a twin pregnancy?

A In a twin pregnancy, there are two babies growing in the same womb. The chances of this happening is 1 in 80. The babies can be in one water bag (uni-ovular or monozygotic twins) and they share the same genes, or in two water bags (dizygotic or binovular twins) and they would be like brothers or sisters.

Q How different is this from a singleton pregnancy?

A In twin pregnancies, all the symptoms of pregnancy tend to be more pronounced. The morning sickness in early pregnancy tends to be worse. So too is the tiredness and dizziness. Low blood haemoglobin level (anaemia) is more common and the patient needs supplements of iron and folic acid. In later pregnancy, joint pains as well as high blood pressure and diabetes are more common. However, of greater significance is that a woman carrying twins tends to deliver earlier before the due date (premature labour). If this happens too early, then survival of the babies would be a problem. To avoid premature labour, a woman with a twin pregnancy should have adequate bed rest and may need to take the drug salbutamol to decrease the incidence of premature labour.

Q What is diabetes and how does it affect the pregnancy?

A In diabetes mellitus the blood sugar level is abnormally high, owing to a deficiency or diminished effect of the hormone insulin. It is characterized by excessive thirst and frequency in passing urine. The hormones of pregnancy makes it easier for diabetes to develop in a pregnant woman. This is especially so in those whose parents have diabetes and in twin pregnancies. If mild, diabetes can be controlled by a careful diet alone. Otherwise, injections of the hormone insulin need to be given. The danger of diabetes is that if it is not well controlled, there is the risk that the baby will die in the womb (stillbirth) or that the mother may become seriously ill from increased acidity in the blood (ketoacidosis).

Q What is pre-eclampsia?

A This is a disease of the pregnant woman which is characterized by two out of three of the following: raised blood pressure, swelling of the legs and protein in the urine. This condition tends to appear in first pregnancies and twin pregnancies. If severe, the patient complains of headache, discomfort in the presence of bright lights and abdominal pain. The blood pressure can be controlled by taking medication and it is important for patients to take their medication regularly. Failure to do so may result in eclampsia, i.e., fits caused by the high blood pressure and this would endanger the life of both mother and baby.

Looking swell, feeling good

Q I am 30 weeks pregnant and notice some prominent veins on my legs. My ankles are also beginning to swell. Are there any exercises which I can do?

A The prominent veins on the legs are varicose veins and are caused by the pressure which the enlarging uterus exerts on the great veins in the pelvis. For varicose veins and swollen ankles, the following measures are helpful and should be done as often as possible. When lying down, raise your legs on pillows so that the ankles are above the level of the heart. Also, with your legs stationary, flex your feet upwards and downwards. Next, move your feet in circular motion clockwise and then anti-clockwise. If the ankle swelling or varicose veins worsen, then you should wear elastic support stockings when you go out and avoid standing for prolonged periods.

Q What about high heels? Should I give them up?

A Yes. The enlarging uterus changes your centre of gravity. This, coupled with slower reflexes during pregnancy, may make you more likely to trip when you wear high heels. Also, your back curves because of the weight of the baby in the womb. This produces greater strain on your back, which high heels tend to aggravate. It is sensible to put your high heels away until after delivery.

Q I experience frequent leg cramps. Is there any exercise which will help?

A Stretching the calf muscles can help alleviate leg cramps. Place your hands against a wall and walk slowly backwards until your heels are lifted off the ground and you feel a stretch in your calf muscles. Hold this position for 30 seconds and then relax. Repeat this a few times.

 I suffer frequent backaches. Is there any exercise to relieve the aches?

Backaches are common in pregnancy, owing to the loosening of ligaments and the increasing weight of the enlarging uterus. You must take care of your posture, especially when carrying out routine tasks. For example, do not bend down to perform chores; instead lower yourself and keep your back straight.

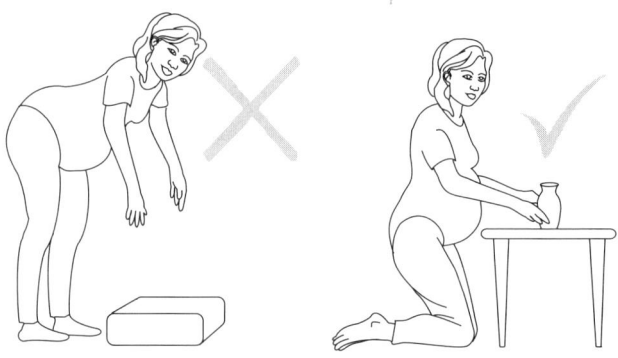

When lifting a heavy load, get into a squatting position, hold the load close to your body and raise it by straightening the legs, all the while keeping your back straight.

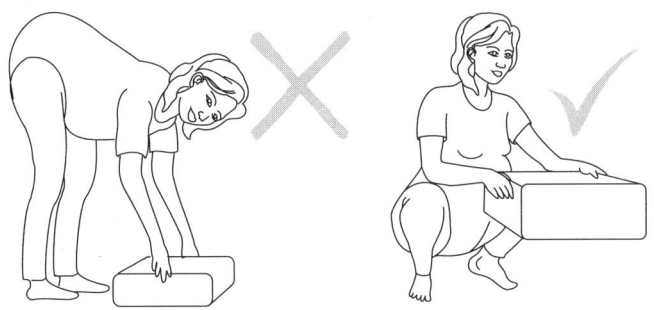

When sitting for prolonged periods, make sure that you have an upright chair with very good back support. Placing a cushion behind the small of your back is useful. Also, make sure that your knees are slightly higher than your hips.

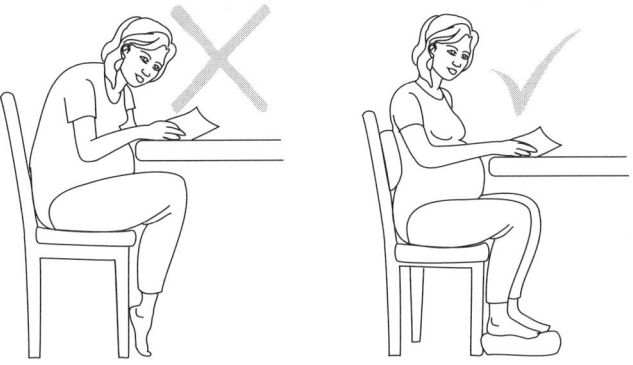

When lying down for prolonged periods, try not to lie flat on your back. The pressure of the large uterus may compress the blood vessels returning blood to the heart. This may in turn cause a reduction of blood flow to the baby and may also make you faint. Instead, lie on your side with a pillow beneath your stomach to give you support and another to support the bent knee of the upper leg.

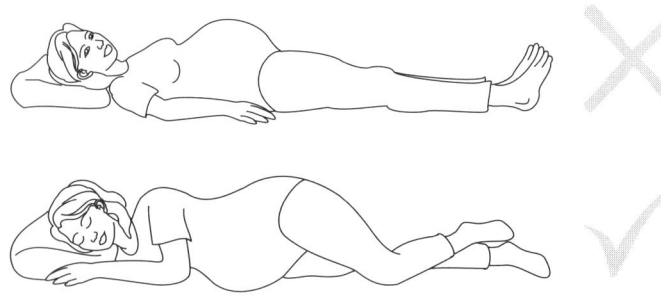

Exercises and breathing techniques for labour

Q Are there any exercises which would help me with labour?

A To prepare for labour, you should keep the large muscles of the back and abdomen in good tone. Firstly, lie on your back with your knees bent. Raise your body while keeping your shoulders and feet on the floor. Hold for 10 seconds and relax. Repeat this a few times.

Next, put one hand under the small of your back. Contract your abdominal muscles and flatten your body onto the back of your hand while tilting your pelvis towards your head. Hold for 10 seconds and relax. Repeat this a few times.

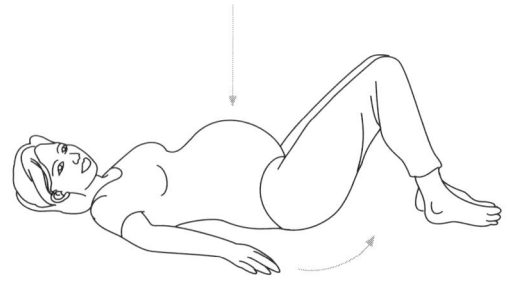

To strengthen the abdominal muscles, lie on your back with your knees bent. Raise your head and place both hands on your knees, hold for 10 seconds and relax. Repeat this a few times.

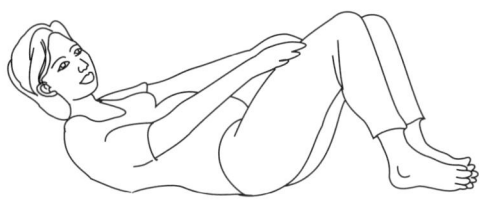

While maintaining your position, part your legs slightly and reach out to touch the right knee. Hold for 10 seconds and relax. Do this for the left knee and repeat this exercise a few times. Avoid doing sit-ups or leg-raising exercises.

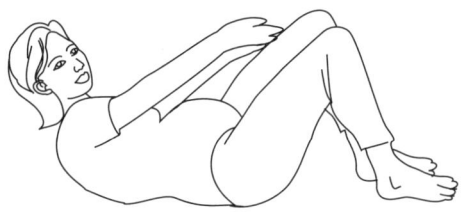

Q Are there any exercises which would help me get into the pushing position for delivery?

A Exercises to loosen the inner thigh muscles would help. Do this by sitting on the floor with your feet close to the body and your soles close together. Press your knees towards the floor, hold for 10 seconds and relax. Repeat this a few times.

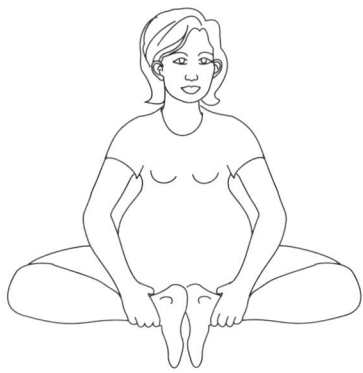

Q   What breathing techniques should I adopt in labour?

A   When you feel the beginning of a contraction, you should slowly take as deep a breath as possible, expanding your whole chest. Then blow out slowly through pursed lips as the pain wears off. In between, you should relax all the muscles of your body.

Alternatively, you may want to practice two levels of breathing. For deep breathing, practice with one hand on your tummy, breathe in deeply through your nose and allow your tummy to expand. After that, blow out slowly through your mouth. Take 10 breaths per minute. This is useful for early contractions.

For shallow breathing, place your hands over your rib cage and breathe in through your nose and allow your chest to expand. Blow out through your mouth and relax. Breathing in this level is quicker and shallower, at 20 to 40 breaths per minute. Shallow breathing is useful for coping with stronger, longer and more frequent contractions.

Remember that for the actual delivery you need to be able to take a deep breath, hold it and push or bear down as hard and as long as possible before breathing in again.

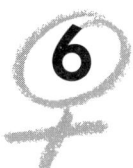

6 Feeding Mum-to-be

Whenever I attend wedding dinners, I will cringe in my seat if a newly expectant mother says, 'I've got to eat for two. I'm pregnant, you know!' If all would-be mothers did that, then soon all the slimming centres would be able to get listed on the main board of the stock exchange.

The truth of the matter is that the quality of the food intake is more important than the quantity. Eating too much of the wrong food only leads to obesity and the excess fat would be difficult to shed later on.

Basic facts about good nutrition

Q Why is it important to have good nutrition in pregnancy?

A It is essential to eat wisely in pregnancy because the baby draws on the mother for its food supply. This is especially so in the second or subsequent pregnancies, when iron or calcium stores may have been used up in the first pregnancy. Good nutrition also prepares the would-be mother for breast feeding and increases the quality and quantity of the breast milk.

What makes a good diet?

A good diet contains all the important nutrients for the developing fetus, in particular protein, folic acid, iron and calcium.

What is the purpose of protein and which food contains it?

Protein is used for building muscles, skin and the body organs like the heart, stomach, kidneys and intestines. Foodstuffs which include high-quality proteins are meats like beef, fish, and chicken, nuts, beans, peas, milk and other dairy products.

What is folic acid? What food contains it?

Folic acid is an important vitamin which is needed for the normal development of the fetus. It is also important for the formation of new blood cells. Folic acid is found in leafy vegetables, orange juice, liver, kidney, dried beans and nuts.

What is the importance of iron in the diet?

Iron is the element essential for the formation of the pigment in red blood cells in both mother and baby. Deficiency of iron in the diet is the commonest cause of anaemia in the pregnant woman. Iron is found in red meat like beef, pork, mutton, liver, nuts and beans. Iron supplements are usually given to the pregnant woman but this sometimes causes constipation and stools which are either blackish or dark green.

Q What about calcium?

A Calcium is important for formation of the baby's bones and teeth. It is also involved in the transmission of nerve impulses and for contraction of the muscles. Calcium is found in milk and dairy products, dark green leafy vegetables like *caixin* and spinach, dried beans and peas, bean curd, small fish with edible bones like *ikan bilis* (anchovies) and sardines.

Q How much weight should I gain in pregnancy?

A The expected weight gain in pregnancy varies considerably, depending on the pre-pregnancy weight. This is measured by the Body Mass Index (BMI) before pregnancy.

$$\text{BMI} = \frac{\text{weight before pregnancy (in kg)}}{\text{height (in m)} \times \text{height (in m)}}$$

Generally, the higher the BMI, the lower the weight gain should be.

Weight gain during pregnancy

If BMI is	Weight status (non-pregnant)	Expected total weight gain (during pregnancy)
less than 20	underweight	12 to 18 kg
20 to less than 25	normal healthy weight	11 to 15 kg
25 to less than 30	mildly overweight	6 to 11 kg
30 or more	very overweight	6 to 9 kg

Weight gain in pregnancy usually begins after the 12th week. The nausea and vomiting in the first 11 weeks can even lead to loss in weight during this period. Weight gain should then be gradual throughout the rest of the pregnancy, with an average of 1 kg every 2 to 3 weeks. The following table is a good guide. Any sudden increase may indicate an excessive amount of water retention, which may herald the onset of pre-eclampsia.

Towards the end of pregnancy, weight gain may actually taper off, but there should be no weight loss. Any loss in weight may indicate that the fetus is not growing well (intrauterine

Recommended average weight gain in pregnancy

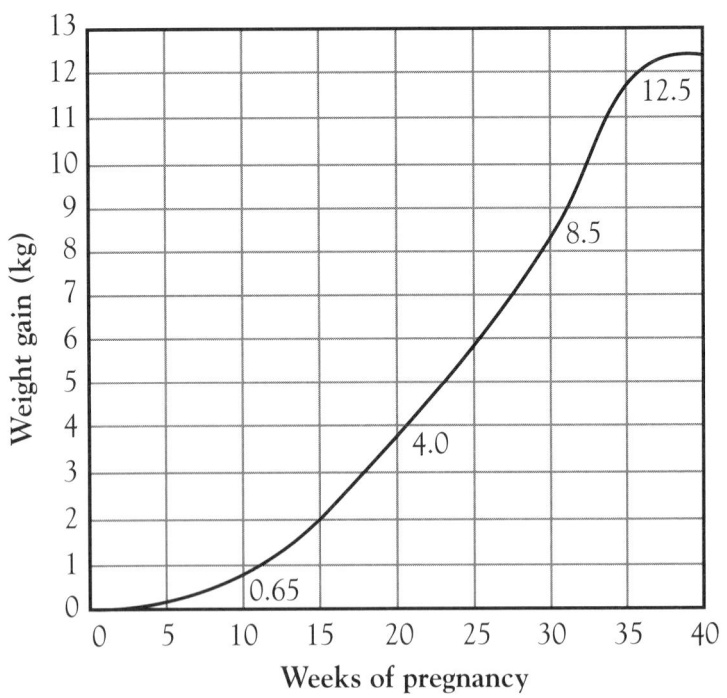

growth retardation). This could mean that the placenta may not be supplying enough nutrients to the baby and may warrant an earlier delivery.

Q In what proportion should the foods be eaten?

A A good general guide can be visually expressed as the 'healthy diet pyramid' as shown in the following figure. In this structure, the foods at the base of the pyramids form the

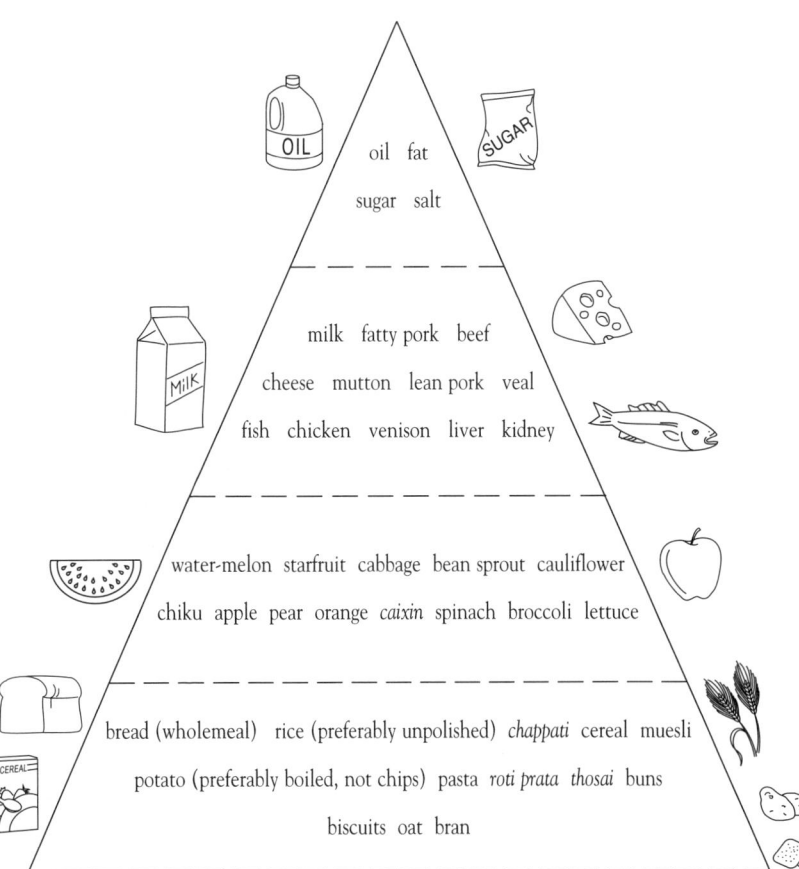

oil   fat
sugar   salt

milk   fatty pork   beef
cheese   mutton   lean pork   veal
fish   chicken   venison   liver   kidney

water-melon   starfruit   cabbage   bean sprout   cauliflower
chiku   apple   pear   orange   *caixin*   spinach   broccoli   lettuce

bread (wholemeal)   rice (preferably unpolished)   *chappati*   cereal   muesli
potato (preferably boiled, not chips)   pasta   *roti prata thosai*   buns
biscuits   oat bran

foundation of the diet or the main source of calories. Hence, they form the bulk of the diet.

Fruits and vegetables form the next level and are important for roughage which prevents constipation, as well as for vitamins and minerals which help fetal growth.

Higher up the pyramid are meats and dairy products like milk. These are important as they are the source of proteins which are essential for growth and development. However, some meats like fatty pork contain high amounts of fats and cholesterol and thus should only be taken in moderation.

At the top of the pyramid are additives like fat, oil, sugar and salt. These, in essence, only provide flavour and hence should be taken as sparingly as possible. In fact, it is possible to get by without any added salt in the food as the small amounts of sodium required in the diet can be found in food in its natural form.

 How much of these foods should be eaten per day?

As a general guide, bread, rice or its alternatives (the base of the pyramid) should be taken in smaller quantities but more frequently – about six servings a day. There should be two servings of fruits and vegetables per day and three servings of meat daily.

 What is one serving of carbohydrate?

One serving is: $^1/_2$ a small bowl of rice or noodles or
       2 slices of bread or
       1 *chappati* or
       1 *roti prata* or
       1 hot dog bun or
       1 cup of breakfast cereal or
       4 plain biscuits

Q What is one serving of fruit?

A This comprises: 1 small apple, pear or orange or
1 wedge of papaya, pineapple,
water-melon or honeydew melon or
6 rambutans or *duku* or
1 banana or
10 grapes

Q What is one serving of vegetables?

A This comprises: 1 cup of cooked leafy vegetables,
e.g. spinach, cabbage or *caixin* or
$1/2$ a cup of cooked non-leafy vegetables,
e.g. carrots, pumpkin, potato,
mushrooms, tomato

It is better to eat more leafy vegetables.

Q What is a serving of meat?

A One serving is: a palm-sized piece of meat, fish or chicken or
5 medium-sized prawns or
2 small *sotong*, cuttlefish, squids or
2 squares of beancurd (*doufu*) or
$1/2$ a cup of cooked lentils, pulses or nuts or
2 glasses of milk or
2 slices of cheese or
2 tablespoons of *ikan bilis*

Q My diet does not sound too palatable!

A It may be lacking in sauces, but the diet above is very
wholesome. The trick is to go for variety in the diet,
especially in the fruits and vegetables.

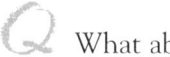 What about fluids?

A pregnant woman needs to drink at least 8 to 10 glasses of fluid per day. Plain water, low-fat milk, fresh fruit or vegetable juices should be taken. Give sweetened soft drinks a wide berth.

Will drinking excessively cause increased swelling in pregnancy?

It is not true that drinking excessive water causes swelling in pregnancy. Water retention in pregnancy is caused mainly by pressure of the enlarging womb or by changes in the composition of the blood in pregnancy. High blood pressure in pregnancy (pre-eclampsia) also causes swelling of the legs.

Is it safe to drink alcohol in pregnancy?

The occasional glass of wine or beer is permissible but excessive consumption of alcohol is bad for the baby as it can cause abnormalities of the heart, limbs and face, as well as growth retardation.

Does eating oranges during pregnancy cause phlegm or jaundice in the baby?

Eating oranges during pregnancy does not predispose the baby to coughs after birth. Also, the only similarity between oranges and a jaundiced baby is the colour! There is definitely no increased tendency to jaundice in the baby.

Q Can I go to the hair-dresser or perm my hair during pregnancy?

A It is safe to have your hair permed during pregnancy. The chemicals are only used on the hair and do not enter the body unless there are open sores on the scalp. The only possible risk is catching the influenza virus in a crowded hair-dressing salon!

7 The Happy Event

The onset of labour is more exciting than an FA cup final.
Joyful anticipation, butterflies in the stomach, pulses racing ..... .
The paint is hardly dry on the wall of the baby's room when it is
time to throw the large pack of nappies into the overnight bag and
head for the hospital.

The onset of labour

Q What are the symptoms of labour?

A These are the onset of regular painful contractions of the womb, discharge of blood mixed with mucus from the vagina (the 'show') and the bursting of the water bag ('leaking liquor'). You should call your obstetrician when any of these three happens.

Q What is false labour?

A Towards the due date, the muscles of the womb tend to be more active. False labour is said to occur when there are contractions of the womb but these are not regular and do not get stronger. False labour is also not accompanied by any 'show'. Examination by the obstetrician would also show the neck of the womb to be closed.

Q How do I differentiate the pain of true labour from that of false labour?

A True labour pains are painful and regular. With the patient lying down on the bed, the husband would be able to observe the womb 'rising up' whenever she feels a contraction.

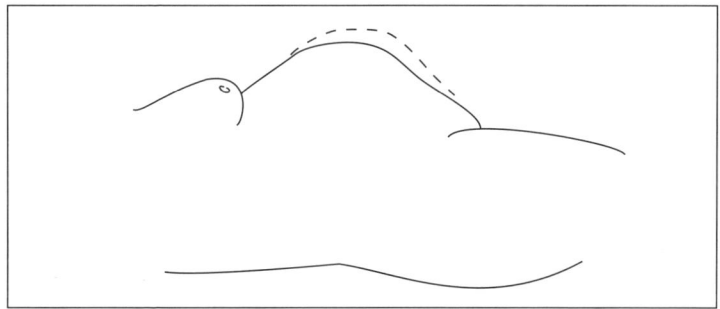

During a contraction, the womb rises visibly.

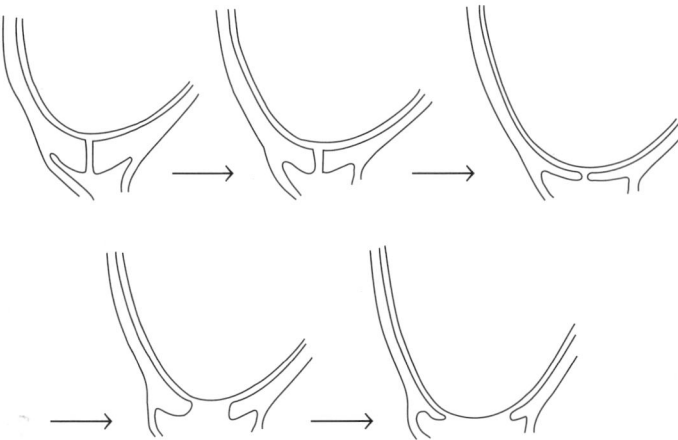

The cervix gradually becomes thin and the opening widens in preparation for delivery of the baby.

They may occur at 10-minute intervals, lasting a few seconds each time. Gradually, they occur once every 5 minutes and then once every 2 minutes, lasting 45 seconds each time. When this occurs, the labour pains are said to be 'established'. At this time, some bloody discharge or show would appear. Examination of the neck of the womb by the obstetrician would confirm it to be opening up.

Q What should I do when true labour begins?

A Having contacted your obstetrician, he would advise you to check into the hospital in which you have been booked. A patient delivering in Singapore needs to bring along her identity card, birth plan, hospital booking slip, investigation results including the blood and ultrasound results, letter from her obstetrician and the marriage certificate (if she intends to use her husband's Medisave account). Do drive carefully as you will not usually deliver so quickly as to make beating red lights necessary. All the hospitals in Singapore are at most an hour away by car (or 2 hours at the most, during peak hours). The rapid delivery of a baby in moving taxis is a very rare occurrence.

On the other hand, do not dawdle either. I had a call one day from a patient who sounded very distressed with her labour pains, so I asked her to head for the hospital immediately. I waited and waited and she finally showed up two-and-a-half hours later with her hair neatly and stylishly done. 'I had to go to the hair-dresser first to have my hair washed and set because my mother-in-law said that I cannot wash my hair for one month after delivery!' she explained.

Q   What happens when I arrive at the hospital?

A   After the documentation and admission processes have been completed, you will be escorted into the labour ward. You may be put in a wheelchair if the labour pains are strong. Once in the labour ward, the midwife will place a plastic identification strap on your wrist and give you a gown to change into. She will then ask you to lie on a bed and then time your contractions. A belt may be strapped over your abdomen for a cardiotocogram (CTG) to be applied. This allows the baby's heart beats and the contractions of the womb to be checked. Your obstetrician or the midwife will then examine you internally to check the opening of the neck of the womb. This procedure will be slightly uncomfortable. It should not hurt but you do need to relax when it is carried out. An enema is then given to empty the bowels so that there will be no contamination of the baby when he is born.

Q   What does it mean when the baby's head is 'engaged'?

A   This is the term used by the obstetrician when the broadest part of the baby's head is at the level of the entrance of the pelvic bone (the pelvic brim).

Engagement is important because in patients where the baby is too big to be delivered normally, the head will usually not be engaged during labour. This is confirmed by examination of the patient's abdomen by the obstetrician. In such a case the baby's head would be found to be above, and not within, the pelvic brim. Engagement of the baby's head usually occurs by the 38th week of pregnancy in first-time pregnancies although it may not occur until the onset of labour in women who have had babies before.

Q How does the baby move through the birth canal?

A The birth canal is formed by the womb and the muscles of the vagina. It is like a tube and can be likened to a drain-pipe bent at right angles so that the opening is at the entrance of the vagina.

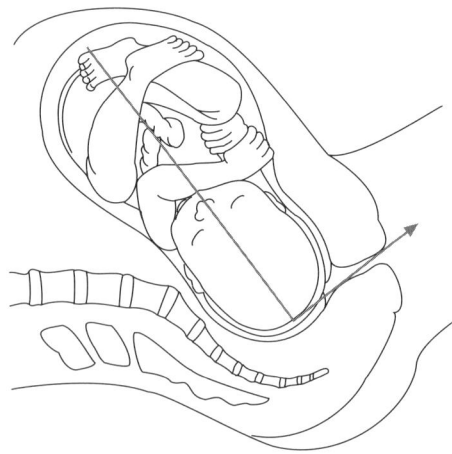

Notice the angle the baby needs to negotiate during delivery

The baby is moved down this 'drain-pipe' by a combination of the contractions of the womb during labour and by the voluntary pushing efforts of the mother when she feels the baby pressing down on her bottom.

The stages of labour

Q How many stages of labour are there?

A There are three stages of labour. The first stage is from the start of the contractions until the neck of the womb (cervix) is fully open, i.e. 10 cm wide. The second stage is from the time the neck of the womb is fully open to the time the baby is born. The third stage is from the time the baby is born until the placenta and membranes of pregnancy are delivered.

Q Will I be able to walk about during the first stage of labour?

A There is a first stage room in the labour ward where patients with uncomplicated labours are allowed to walk about if they wish. The advantage of walking is that it is a form of distraction therapy which serves to alleviate somewhat the pain of labour. Also, it helps the descent of the baby's head into the birth canal. The disadvantage, however, is that it makes it more difficult to monitor the baby's heartbeat. This is important as problems with the baby (fetal distress) may arise unexpectedly during labour.

Q How long will it be before the baby is born?

A The duration of labour is somewhat variable. In first-time labours, once the cervix has opened to 3 cm (the active phase of labour), further opening usually progresses at 1 cm per hour until the neck of the womb is fully opened to 10 cm. It then takes another hour for the baby to be delivered. To put it differently, if a woman who is pregnant for the first time enters the labour room and her obstetrician finds her cervix to be opened to 5 cm, then it should take 5 hours for the rest of the first stage and another hour for the second stage. In all, it will be 6 hours before the baby is delivered.

For women who have delivered before, the duration of labour is usually much shorter. The whole process from the first stage to the end of the second stage, when the baby is born, may be

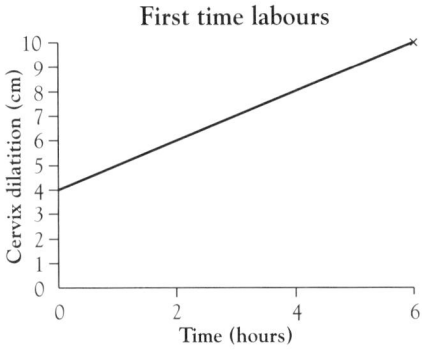

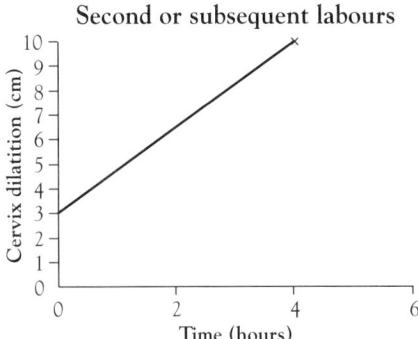

Subsequent labours progress more quickly than first time labours although the time may not exactly be halved.

only an hour. This is usually so for women who have had short labours before.

There is this true story of a patient who delivered on the ambulance trolley en route to the labour ward of a government hospital in Singapore. She was very embarrassed and apologized profusely to the nurses over the mess she had made. The nurses were very understanding and tried to comfort her, saying, 'No, please don't worry. It's really alright. Why, 2 years ago, there was a lady who even delivered in the carpark of the hospital!' To which the patient replied, 'Yes, that was also me!'

Although such stories are very rare, I usually tell patients who have had short labours before to go to the hospital early. Here is a first-person account of a patient who had a normal delivery:

Sweet slumber lasted until 12.15 a.m. that night. Rude awakening came as a wet, cold feeling. I sat up and found myself sitting in a pool of water. Did our water-bed spring a leak? As I woke my husband up, I felt fluid flowing out of my lower body. It dawned on our sleepy minds that it was the obstetrician we needed, not the repairman!

Baby had decided to spring a surprise on us – Baby was not due for another 2 weeks! Surprised we may have been, but we were well prepared. Armed with the bag we had earlier packed for my hospital stay, the breathing exercises we had learnt in the antenatal classes and a prayer, we headed for hospital. We had our roles clearly in our heads – Hubby's job was to get us to hospital safely and my job was to handle the labour coolly and calmly. Once there, he would do all that supportive husbands do and I would, well, handle my labour coolly and calmly.

Much easier said and planned than done, we soon found out. While Hubby concentrated on his driving, IT – labour pain – struck me. I did my best with the breathing exercises, trying not to distract him. The pain was worse than any I had experienced before but I dealt with it stoically and, might I add, heroically.

At the hospital, the midwife examined me promptly and found that my cervix was dilated to 1 cm. So much pain and 9 cm more to go. I was hooked up to a machine to monitor the contractions and Baby's heartbeats. In the next bed was another woman with a 4-cm dilation. She was not in the throes of pain; she was chatting happily with her husband! Some people were just born to go through life's experiences more heroically than others, I reasoned to myself.

The pain got steadily and unbelievably worse. I clung to – no, I wrung – Hubby's hand. That did nothing to lessen my pain (probably inflicted some on his hand). In my frustration, I sent him out of the room. Then I missed him terribly. Where was he when I needed him? He came back, explaining that he had gone for a walk. Fine time to pick for a walk. I wrung his hand some more. Still no relief. Hubby hovered around and then decided to read the papers and help himself to some biscuits. I unleashed all my pent-up irritation and frustration. I was nowhere near the cool and calm woman I had planned to be but I was beyond caring.

When the dilation reached 5 cm, I was given an injection to help relieve the pain and, I half suspect, to relieve Hubby's suffering as well. It made a world of difference. I was also comforted to learn that Hubby had got our friends to pray for me. I dozed off and when I woke up, my cervix was almost fully dilated.

I was transferred to the labour ward. I felt the urge to push many times but had to hold back until the cervix was fully dilated. The time came, I pushed only twice and soon after, my smiling obstetrician placed Baby Samuel on my chest. With a little help, labour need not be a trying time at all, I had found out. And Baby Samuel, our priceless reward, made it all worthwhile.

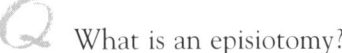

What is an episiotomy?

An episiotomy is a small cut made at the lower part of the vagina to allow for the baby's head to be delivered.

Is it always necessary?

It is usually necessary for patients delivering their first babies as the skin of the vagina is rather tight because it has not been stretched by previous deliveries. If an episiotomy is not made, then the lower part of the vagina may tear naturally during childbirth and this tear may reach the anus

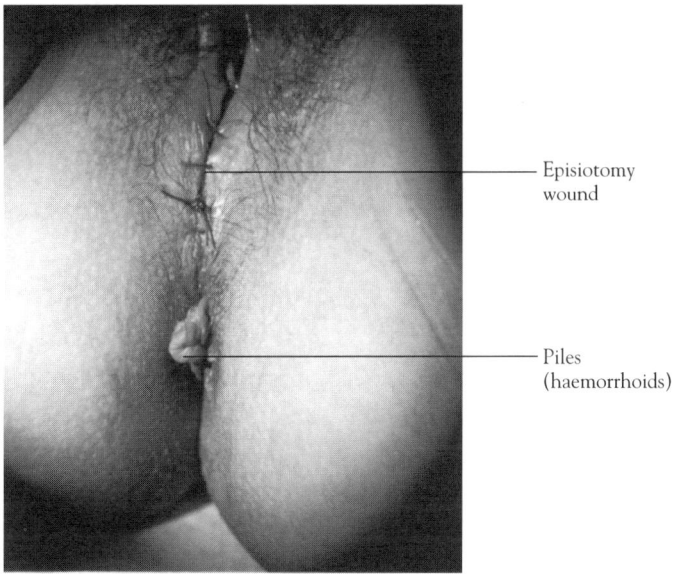

Episiotomy
wound

Piles
(haemorrhoids)

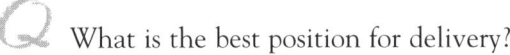

The episiotomy wound is stitched together after the labour is over.
Notice the piles, which commonly occurs as a result of pregnancy and labour.

behind and affect the patient's bowel movements later. Also, a clean cut is easier to stitch and therefore would heal better than a jagged tear. It may not be necessary to perform episiotomies even in first labours unless the situation warrants it. For second or third deliveries, stretching of the skin of the lower vagina is usually sufficient to allow delivery to take place without an episiotomy.

Q What is the best position for delivery?

A There is no hard and fast rule here. Most patients find it easiest to deliver the baby lying on their back at a slight upward tilt. They have their legs drawn up, with their hands grasping their ankles for leverage.

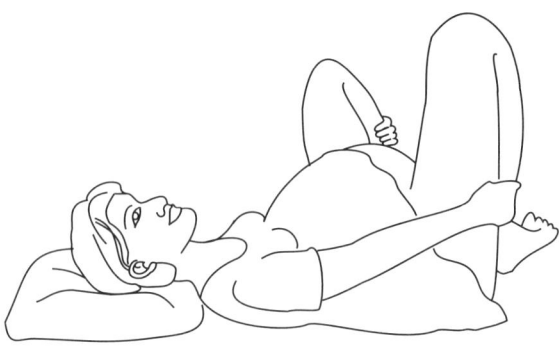

In this position , they are encouraged to hold their breath and bear down whenever they feel a contraction. If necessary, the midwife would help a little by pressing on the top of the womb (applying fundal pressure).

Some patients prefer to deliver their baby in the squatting position but this has a disadvantage – it makes it difficult for the obstetrician to protect the lower vagina. Hence ugly and severe tears to the anus may occur if the patient pushes hard with strong contractions.

Q Can my husband be present during my delivery?

A It is good for husbands to be present to share in the joy of the birth process. They also play an important supporting role by being at the bedside. By chatting with the patient, he can help distract her and the pain of labour becomes less severe. I had a patient once who played Scrabble with her husband throughout her 8-hour labour and beat him just before the baby was delivered!

However, some husbands are squeamish and do not take the sight or smell of blood well. In such an instance, he should be advised to stand just outside if he feels ill. Last year I had a 19-year-old father who fainted and hit his head on the floor after the baby was delivered. Both mother and baby were fit to go home after 3 days but the father, who had a concussion, had to stay 2 extra days!

Q What forms of pain relief are available for the woman in labour?

A Numerous methods are available. Simple breathing techniques, injections of a pain-relieving drug, inhaling nitrous oxide and epidural pain relief are the more commonly used methods.

Q How can breathing be used to lessen pain?

A Controlled breathing techniques are extremely useful in lessening pain. The patient feels the start of a contraction and takes a deep breath in. She then holds her breath and blows out slowly as the contraction wears off. Many of my patients are able to go through a large part of the first stage or even the whole birth process just by controlled breathing.

Q I have an extremely low pain threshold. What if breathing techniques do not work?

A Then a pain-relieving injection of pethidine is given into the side of the thigh. This is repeated 4 to 6 hours later if you require further pain relief.

Q What is pethidine? Does it produce any side-effects?

A Pethidine is a form of morphine. Labour is one of the times when you can consume morphine without getting into trouble with the law! Pethidine injections lessen pain and gives the patient a mild euphoria (feeling of happiness).

However, it also causes drowsiness, nausea and vomiting in some women. These side-effects can be controlled by other drugs which stop nausea and vomiting. Pethidine, if given too close to delivery, may affect the baby's breathing immediately after birth but this effect can be reversed by giving a drug called naloxone to stimulate the baby's breathing. Before giving pethidine, the obstetrician or midwife would examine the patient to see whether the neck of the womb if fully open. If so, then pethidine may be withheld and another form of pain relief, like nitrous oxide gas, given instead.

Q What is nitrous oxide?

A Nitrous oxide is a pain-relieving gas and is otherwise known as laughing gas. The patient holds a rubber mask and takes a deep breath of the gas mixture when she finds the pain coming on. It is especially useful towards the end of the first stage of labour, when the baby would be born soon. This is because unlike pethidine, it does not cause breathing problems in the newborn.

Q What if pethidine or nitrous oxide still does not work?

A Then we bring out the heavy artillery. Epidural pain relief (epidural analgesia) involves the insertion of a very thin plastic tube into the back of the patient while she lies on her side with her legs drawn up. This is performed by the anaesthetist (not the obstetrician, thank God!), who is a specialist doctor trained in relieving pain. The end of this tube lies in a space just outside the spinal cord from which large nerves emerge. An injection of an anaesthetic agent through this tube will numb the nerves which carry pain impulses from the womb.

Q Is the epidural dangerous?

A Properly given by a good anaesthetist, epidural analgesia is a very safe and effective form of pain relief in labour. Occasionally, problems may arise. The patient may shiver and there may be a sudden fall in blood pressure, which may cause problems for the fetus. This can be reversed by running a drip solution rapidly to increase the patient's blood volume.

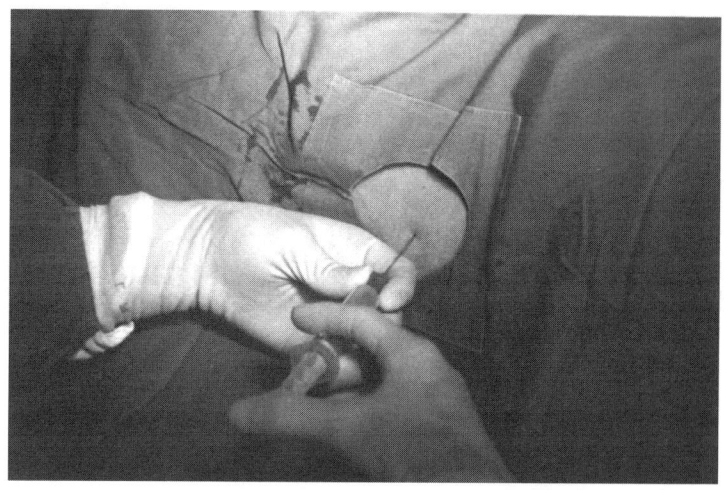

Administering the epidural

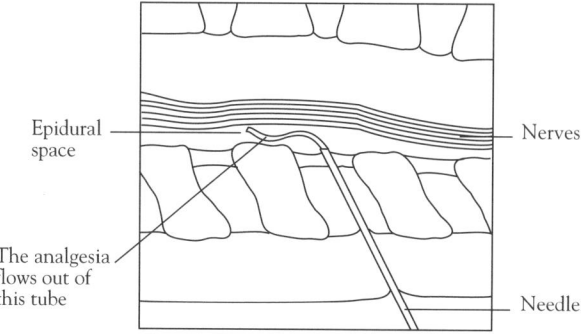

Epidural space

Nerves

The analgesia flows out of this tube

Needle

With an epidural, the patient's ability to push may be impaired as the anaesthetic drug may also block the nerves supplying the muscles of the lower vagina. In rare instances, backache after the procedure, sometimes lasting a few weeks to months, may occur. Rarer still is the occasional report of weakness or even paralysis of the legs following an epidural. These complications may sound frightening but if a patient requires pain relief, then she should take it. Labour should be a pleasurable experience as it heralds the birth of your baby. As doctors, we would strive to abolish pain and make labour as pleasant and memorable as possible.

Q Is there any other form of pain relief?

A Hypnosis and transcutaneous electrical nerve stimulation (TENS) have been tried. In TENS, a small electrical gadget with wires coming out of it is used. At the ends of the wires are electrodes. The patient attaches the electrodes to the skin of her abdomen. With the device switched on, intermittent electrical impulses are released and the patient feels a tingling sensation. This is useful for mild pain and may work sometimes in advanced labour. It has no side-effects whatsoever on the fetus.

Assisted delivery

Q What if the mother is unable to push to deliver the baby?

A This may happen, especially with an epidural. The obstetrician may then help the patient by using vacuum delivery or forceps.

Q What is a vacuum delivery?

A In a vacuum delivery, the obstetrician helps the patient by applying a rubber or metal cup over the baby's head when it is still in the vagina. A electrical pump then creates suction pressure and the obstetrician pulls, with the patient pushing, during a contraction. This then brings about the delivery of the baby's head. The rest of the baby soon follows.

Applying the vacuum cup

Making the episiotomy and using a rubber tubing to create a vacuum (negative pressure)

Delivering the baby's head using the vacuum cup

What is the danger of a vacuum delivery?

This is usually very safe. Occasionally, there may be damage to the baby's scalp where the cup is attached or the formation of a small blood clot outside the skull bone. These usually soon subside on their own.

 What is a forceps delivery?

In a forceps delivery, the obstetrician uses a pair of metal tongs to hold and gently pull out the baby's head to help the mother during delivery. It is used when the mother is unable to push out the baby on her own as when she is on an epidural or when the baby is in distress, as shown by a fall in the baby's heart beat.

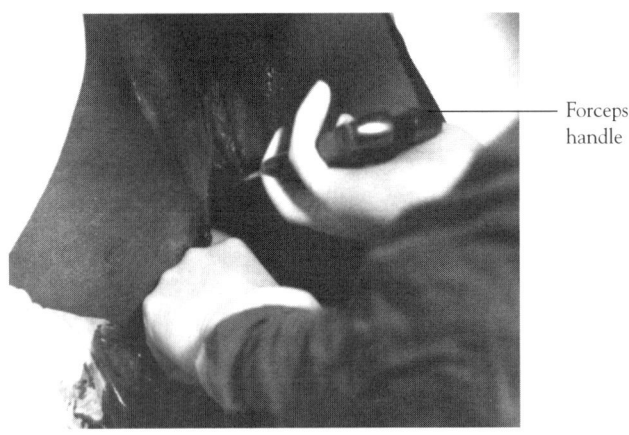

Forceps handle

Delivery with the aid of forceps

 Is there any danger in a forceps delivery?

 Again, this is generally very safe if done properly. Sometimes, the blades of the forceps leave marks on the baby's face but these soon disappear. In rare instances, more serious damage to the head, with internal bleeding, may occur. As such, forceps are used in situations when delay in delivery would result in even graver consequences.

Q What if the baby needs to be delivered urgently and the vacuum or forceps is unable to bring on delivery?

A Then a emergency Caesarean section needs to be done. This involves shaving the patient, putting up a drip and quickly moving her into the operating theatre, where the anaesthetist would give the patient a general anaesthesia. If the patient is already under an epidural, then the Caesarean section can be done under the influence of the epidural, with the patient still awake. A horizontal cut about 10 cm long is made at the upper border of the pubic hair line. Through this incision the baby is delivered. Here is a first-person account from a patient who underwent a Caesarean section:

It had been 39 weeks and my husband had taken to calling me an over-weight hippopotamus. My weight during the last 2 weeks had decreased (not that my husband noticed it) and my obstetrician worried that my placenta might be weakening. He advised that I have my labour induced.

At 8 p.m. on Tuesday, I settled into the hospital room, with Mother's chicken soup in my tummy. It would give me strength for my labour, she had promised. I was hooked up to a machine that monitored the fetus' heartbeats and my contractions. The nurse inserted a tablet into my vagina to get the contractions going. Over the next hour, my husband pored studiously over the chart from the machine and announced, with an air of expertise, that there were no contractions. Man and machine having both confirmed what I already knew, we settled down for the night.

At 5 a.m. on Wednesday, the nurse woke me up for my shower and a meagre breakfast. I was wired up to the machine again. Man and machine now tell me I have small contractions. Now that was news – I barely felt a thing! My obstetrician breezed in, put me on a drip to further stimulate the contractions and burst my waterbag. The gush of water lessened to a trickle and my dilatation was about 3 – 4 cm.

Noon came and went, and still no sign of Baby. The contractions got stronger but my husband (What would I have done without him?) reminded me of the breathing exercises we learnt at our antenatal classes. The technique helped and I was confident I could go through the labour without additional help, strong woman that I was.

It was afternoon and the contractions have got the better of me. The nurse helpfully offered me a pethidine injection, which I bravely dismissed … at first. Half an hour of contractions later, I meekly gave in to her suggestion. Relief was almost instantaneous although it was supposed to have taken effect after about half an hour. Two hours later, the pains were back and unbearable. I abandoned all sense of decorum and hollered for an epidural.

My obstetrician came by again. I was only 5 – 6 cm dilated and my husband discussed the possibility of a C-section with him.

Dinner time came … and went. I was running a fever and beginning to feel woozy. The nurse gave me a glass of glucose to sip. The nurse for the night shift came by. She found that I was almost fully dilated and, together with my husband, encouraged me to push whenever I felt a contraction. The end was in sight!

However, 9.30 p.m. came and still no baby! Mother's nutritious chicken soup was all used up. I was nauseated and shivering violently. My obstetrician came by and we all agreed that a C-section was in order. From that point, things happened at lightning speed.

I was wheeled into the operating theatre and my husband had to wait outside. As I was already on the epidural, the anaesthetist only needed to top it up. I did not need a general anaesthesia. I could no longer hold back my nausea so I threw up and felt much better after that. I could not feel my obstetrician cutting up my tummy but I heard the clink and the clank of the instruments he used. I felt the tugging and pulling. Voila! Baby cried.

The nurse wrapped her up and placed the screaming bundle on my chest. My bundle of joy gave me her big wide-eyed look and I knew what it was to feel this all-encompassing maternal love. I only vaguely remember my obstetrician stitching me up.

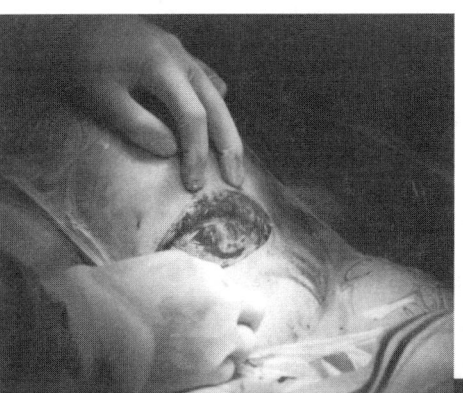

At the start, a cut is made in the abdomen.

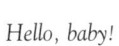

Hello, baby!

8

And Baby Makes Three

Definition of a baby:

A loud noise at one end and no sense of responsibility at the other.
attributed to Ronald Knox (1888–1957)

Most of us look at babies in a far more romantic light. Whichever way we choose to look at them, the truth is, once baby comes home, life will never be the same again.

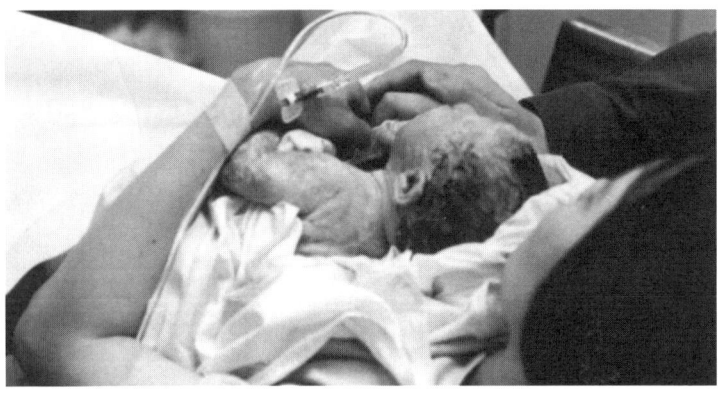

Breast feeding

Q What are the benefits of breast feeding?

A The benefits of breast feeding for both mother and baby are well established. For the mother, it brings about a faster recovery of the womb to the non-pregnant state.

Women who breast feed their babies have a lower incidence of breast cancer (the commonest cancer in females) in later life.

Breast feeding also enhances the baby's health. Antibodies to many infectious diseases are passed from the mother to the baby through the breast milk. These antibodies would prevent the newborn baby from getting many illnesses like influenza for at least for 2 to 3 months until the baby develops his own immunity. Breast milk is also always at the right temperature and contains no bacteria. The breast-fed baby is also less likely to develop asthma, infections of the bowel, allergic diseases and even serious conditions like leukaemia in later life.

Among the other benefits of breast feeding is the establishment of the mother–baby bond. The close physical and emotional contact during the many hours of feeding is perhaps the most important factor in forging this relationship. The mother is personally involved in nurturing her infant and thereby feels a sense of accomplishment. The baby is accorded a close and comfortable physical relationship with his mother and this gives the baby a sense of security and a feeling of being loved.

My breasts are small and the nipples are inverted. Can I still breast feed?

The size of the breasts has no bearing on the ability to breast feed. It is the hormone, prolactin, which is produced by the brain after delivery, that causes the enlargement of the milk ducts and the release of colostrum and then milk. This process is not dependant on the size of the breast. Inverted nipples can be made to protrude by using a nipple shield. This is a soft plastic cup which is placed over the inverted nipple. Gentle pressure on the nipple shield would cause most cases of inverted nipples to protrude normally. If this fails, then breast feeding is still possible by allowing the baby to suckle or by expressing the milk. Milk can be expressed either manually or by using an electrical pump.

Q What is colostrum?

A Colostrum is a thin, slightly yellow turbid fluid rich in protein and fat. This is secreted by the breasts towards the end of pregnancy and immediately after the delivery of the baby. It also contains antibodies from the mother which protect the baby against various diseases. Colostrum is 8.6 per cent protein, 2.3 per cent fat, 3.2 per cent carbohydrate and 85.6 per cent water.

Q How exactly is breast feeding carried out?

A One way is to feed the baby at fixed intervals throughout the day and night. The other way is demand feeding, which is to feed the baby as and when he cries.

First, the nipples are gently cleaned with a CLEAN warm moist hand towel which is then sent to the wash. The mother is seated comfortably on a low chair with good back support. The head of the baby is then cradled in the crook of the arm and the baby's mouth guided to the nipple. The baby would immediately 'latch on' and begin sucking vigorously. Some tenderness of the nipples would be felt especially by first-time mothers. Hence feeding should not be longer than 5 minutes on either side. By this time, the breast on the feeding side should be soft and the other side would be dripping with milk. The mother should then switch sides and repeat this until either the baby is fully fed and falls asleep or yells his head off as there is inadequate milk.

For the first week before breast feeding is fully established, it may be necessary to supplement breast feeding with the bottle after each feed. However, this soon becomes unnecessary, with the baby feeding solely on breast milk.

The fully fed baby is then made to sit upright, with the thumb and forefinger of one hand supporting the floppy head and the palm of the other hand stroking the baby's back upwards to elicit a burp. After this is over, the baby is gently laid down on his front on a firm mattress while the mother cleans her nipples with a clean damp hand towel. This towel is then sent to the wash and a lanolin-based cream applied onto the nipples.

Q My lower tummy hurts every time I breast feed. Is this normal?

A During breast feeding, there will be some low abdominal pain as a hormone (oxytocin) released by the brain during breast feeding causes contractions of the womb.

Q After a few days of breast feeding, my nipples are cracked and painful. What can I do?

A Cracked nipples are common during the first week of breast feeding because during this time, the milk flow has not yet been established. This results in the baby sucking vigorously to obtain sufficient breast milk. Excessive washing of the nipples with a strong soap also contributes to cracked nipples. The skin of the nipple secretes its own natural oils and excessive washing with soap removes the oils, leading to cracking of the skin. Treatment is by applying a lanolin-based cream 3 times a day.

Also, the baby should not be allowed to suck for too long on the same side. It is usually advisable to let the baby suckle for 5 minutes on each breast and if the baby is still hungry after half an hour of breast feeding, supplement the feed with bottled milk until full breast feeding is established. Before this happens, breast feeding on empty breasts only causes the baby to be frustrated and cry incessantly, the mother to feel pain and the father to despair.

Q What are the causes of painful breasts?

A The commonest cause of painful breasts is engorgement caused by accumulated milk, usually during the first week after delivery. On examination, the breasts are hard and tender with swollen veins visible on its surface. There may be a mild fever. The treatment for engorged breasts is to empty the breasts of the accumulated milk by feeding the baby or by expressing the milk manually or by using an electric pump. If this fails to provide relief, warm compresses and a tablet of bromocriptine can be given to decrease milk production temporarily. It is important to treat engorged breasts promptly or else the accumulated milk may become infected, leading to breast infection (mastitis).

Q What are the signs of mastitis?

A In this condition, the breasts are painful and swollen, with an area of redness usually near the nipple. This red area is more tender than the rest of the breast. The patient may have a fever with chills and shivering. Early infection of the breasts can be successfully treated with antibiotics and breast feeding need be only temporarily withheld. Any delay in treatment could cause the area to be inflamed and pus to form. In this situation, milk production would need to be stopped and breast feeding terminated. High doses of the appropriate antibiotic would then arrest the infection but if there is a collection of pus, then an operation would be required to drain it.

Q What sort of diet is good for breast feeding?

A A breast-feeding mother needs to drink a large amount of fluid daily. This can take the form of water, tea or a lightly flavoured drink with honey. A woman who is dehydrated will be unable to produce sufficient amounts of breast milk. Drinking fresh cow's milk is important as this provides the necessary nutrients. Fish, chicken, beef and mutton would supply the necessary proteins. Calcium supplements in the form of tablets are necessary to replace calcium stores in the body.

Recipes for the new mum

Given on the following pages are four recipes of herbal tonics which are popular for the post-delivery period. They are equally useful after miscarriages and should be taken 2 to 3 times weekly for 1 to 2 months after the event. The next four recipes do not require herbs but are equally popular for the immediate postnatal period.

Tonic for general weakness and exhaustion
(contributed by loss of blood):
bazhen soup

Tonic for dizziness:
You need:

10 g *tianma*	10 g *danggui*
10 g *baizhi*	10 g *heshouwu*
10 g *chuanxiong*	10 g *huangqi*

150 g meat or half a chicken
3 bowls of water

Put all the ingredients into a pot and boil for 3 to 4 hours.

Tonic for intolerance of cold:
3 g Korean ginseng
10 g quizi
100 g meat
1 bowl of water

Put the ingredients into a double-boiler and boil for 2 hours.

Tonic for aches in the loins:

10 g *duzhong*	10 g *dangshen*
10 g *bajitian*	10 g *qizi*
10 g *huangqi*	

150 g meat or half a chicken
3 bowls of water

Put all the ingredients into a pot and boil for 3 to 4 hours.

Chicken in sesame oil

You need:

1 chicken drumstick, de-boned and cut into bite-sized
   pieces
3 tablespoons of sesame oil
5 slices of ginger
1 clove of garlic, chopped
   pinch of salt

1. Heat the pan and put in the sesame oil.
2. Put in the garlic and stir-fry.
3. Add in the ginger and stir-fry until fragrant and slightly brown.
4. Put in the chicken and salt. Stir-fry for a few minutes until the chicken is cooked.
5. Serve hot, with steamed rice.

Fried chicken with pepper

You need:

1 chicken drumstick, de-boned and cut into 2
1 tablespoon of sugar
2 tablespoons of coarsely ground pepper
1 tablespoon of dark soya sauce
oil for frying

1. Marinade the chicken with the sugar, pepper and soya sauce for 10 minutes.
2. Heat the pan and put in the oil.
3. Fry the chicken, turning the pieces over to brown both sides.
4. Serve hot, with steamed rice.

Double-boiled black chicken with pepper

You need:
1 black chicken, skinned
5 slices of ginger
3 tablespoons of coarsely ground pepper
1 teaspoon of salt

1. Put all the ingredients into a double-boiler.
2. Add boiling water to cover the chicken.
3. Double-boil on medium heat for $1^1/_2$ to 2 hours.
4. Serve hot, with steamed rice.

Wheat noodle soup *(mianxian tang)*

You need:
1 bundle of *mianxian*, blanched
5 slices of fresh pig's liver
5 pieces of pig's kidney (optional)
5 pieces of minced pork balls
5 bite-sized pieces of *ikan kurau*
2 bowls of water

Seasoning:
1 tablespoon of cooking oil
2 slices of ginger
1 teaspoon of chopped garlic
1 teaspoon of sliced shallots
1 teaspoon of light soya sauce
1 tablespoon of sesame oil
1 teaspoon of chopped coriander leaves (optional)
   pinch of salt
dash of pepper

Marinade for kidney:
1 tablespoon of brandy

Marinade for *ikan kurau*:
1 teaspoon of cornflour
1 teaspoon of light soya sauce
dash of pepper

1. Clean the kidney thoroughly and soak it in lightly salted water to remove the smell. Wash it, drain away the water and marinade it in brandy.
2. Marinade the fish in the cornflour, soya sauce and pepper.
3. Heat the wok. Add the cooking oil, then the ginger, shallots and garlic. Stir-fry until slightly brown.
4. Add in the water, soya sauce and salt.
5. Put in the pork balls and let the soup boil for a few minutes.
6. Next add the fish, liver and kidney.
7. Bring the soup to the boil and add the *mianxian*.
8. Serve in a bowl. Add sesame oil, pepper and coriander leaves.

Q I would like to breast feed but am working full time. What do you suggest?

A Where there is a will, there is a way. Breast feeding will be established during the period of maternity leave during which time milk should be practically dripping from the other breast at the time of breast feeding. Milk from the dripping breast can be expressed into a sterile bottle. Cap the bottle and label it with the date and time at which it was expressed.

Store it in the freezer immediately. A stockpile of milk is thus built up.

Upon resuming work, you need to feed the baby in the morning before leaving for work. Subsequent feeds are then carried out using the stored milk. The bottle that is stored first is used up first after it is warmed in a water bath. Upon return from work, breast feed the baby again and then as often as necessary. It is important that you get adequate rest and intake of fluids so that the quantity of breast milk is maintained.

The road to recovery

Q What other condition can cause fever during this period?

A Fever, especially with foul-smelling vaginal discharge and tenderness over the lower abdomen would indicate infection of the inner surface of the womb (endometritis) or even the surrounding tissue (pelvic cellulitis or pelvic inflammatory disease). This can happen because there is a large raw surface in the womb and bacteria from the anus close by can easily cause infection. A sample of the discharge is sent to the laboratory for confirmation of the diagnosis and identification of the bacteria. Appropriate antibiotic treatment is then given and the fever should subside within a week.

Q I have difficulty controlling my urination after delivery. Why is this so?

A The muscles controlling the opening of the bladder are stretched during the course of delivery. This stretching causes a certain amount of looseness so that when pressure is exerted on the bladder, e.g. when sneezing, coughing or lifting heavy weights, urine leaks out of the bladder. This condition is usually only temporary and full recovery would take place after a few weeks.

Q   Is pain on passing urine normal?

A   A slight smarting sensation over the vaginal wound is common and is due to the slightly acidic urine irritating the episiotomy. However, low abdominal pain, especially a smarting sensation where the urine stream comes out of the bladder is abnormal and could indicate infection of the bladder (cystitis). This is extremely likely if there is blood in the urine (haematuria). Cystitis can be checked by examining the urine under a microscope. It is confirmed when bacteria and plenty of white blood cells show up. Treatment with the appropriate antibiotics, e.g. nalidixic acid, is usually effective.

Q   My stitches still hurt after 2 weeks. Is this normal?

A   The pain from the vaginal tear should lessen over the course of 2 weeks. Pain may still be felt then but any increase in the amount of pain, especially if its associated with a yellow to green foul-smelling pus, indicates infection of the wound.

Q   How can this be treated?

A   A course of antibiotics, together with an antiseptic solution wash for the stitches, would generally be all that is needed to overcome the infection. For pain relief, a sitz bath is useful. The patient puts 3 tablespoons of salt into a basin half-filled with warm water and sits in the solution for 10 minutes 2 to 3 times a day.

Q After delivery, there are some lumps like flesh around my anus. What are these?

A These are commonly piles (haemorrhoids) which develop because of the strong pushing by the mother in the course of childbirth. These are not serious and usually improve on their own. If troublesome, a cream, or a tablet which is inserted into the anus (anal suppository) is used. Rarely do the piles become very painful and tender (thrombosed piles) and for these, an operation to remove them may be necessary.

Q How long does vaginal bleeding last after delivery?

A Usually vaginal bleeding after delivery (lochia) lasts for 3 weeks. For the first week, the bleeding is usually red. It gradually turns to brown and by the third week, it is yellow.

Q Is heavy bleeding a week after giving birth normal?

A Heavy bleeding, especially with clots, a week after delivery (secondary post-partum haemorrhage) is abnormal. This is usually caused by infection of small pieces of placenta retained after delivery. Bleeding may be profuse and the patient needs immediate medical attention as fainting and loss of consciousness may result. If necessary, she would be hospitalized and an intravenous drip set up to replace blood and to give antibiotics. If the bleeding persists, then the patient needs to be brought into the operating theatre where the womb is cleaned out with a D & C procedure. Here is a first-person account:

It was 10 days after I had given birth to my beautiful baby. I was happily feeding her when I felt a warm gush down my legs. I looked down in time to see a large clot slide down my ankle. Fresh blood followed. I was petrified. I went to the toilet to clean up but the bleeding continued. I called my husband, who contacted my obstetrician. He asked us to go to the nearest hospital immediately, where he would meet us.

As we arrived, I could still feel blood running down my legs and I was beginning to feel faint. The lights above me began to swim as I felt my obstetrician give me a painful injection into my left hand. He examined me internally and soon I heard him explain that I would have to be brought into the operating theatre for a D & C. The operating theatre was a scary place with everybody wearing a cap and a gown. There I was placed on a hard metal table. An anaesthetist put this black mask on me and I passed out.

When I awoke, I was back in the ward. My bottom felt sore. My obstetrician came by and showed me some fleshy pieces in a glass bottle. He explained that I had an abnormal placenta – there was an extra portion which got infected and was removed. The next day, my bleeding was much less and I was allowed to go home.

Q Should I take alcoholic drinks after delivery? Does this pose any danger?

A Alcohol is useful in colder climates as it causes an increase in body warmth. However, excessive consumption of alcohol can, in theory, cause an increase in vaginal bleeding. This is because it relaxes the muscles of the womb; contraction of the muscles of the womb is necessary for blood loss to cease.

Q I am a Muslim. What traditional medicine can I use after delivery?

A Many of my Muslim patients use a mixture called *param* to clean their skin. They also apply a mud-coloured mixture called *pilis* on their foreheads. To aid in shrinkage of the abdomen, they use a mixture of lime and other substances as a body wrap.

As for their diet, they usually eat fish, chicken and vegetables either boiled or steamed. Soups are cooked with ginger and garlic, which are believed to aid in the digestion. Too much spicy food is avoided as this may cause abdominal discomfort.

Q Is there any harm in using traditional medication?

A Traditional medication which is applied externally is generally harmless. That which is consumed for short periods is also safe but such medication should not be taken in excess. This is because the medicinal chemicals in herbs or roots are not scientifically quantified. Hence there is a risk of overdosage if large quantities are taken over prolonged periods.

Q The calf of my left leg hurts badly especially when I squeeze it. Is this serious?

A Muscular pains after delivery are common. However, pain in one leg with tenderness on deep pressure may indicate blockage of the veins of the leg by a blood clot (deep vein thrombosis). This is a serious condition as the blood clot may dislodge itself and find its way into the large blood vessels of the lungs . Blockage of these vessels (pulmonary embolism) is very serious as it may cause death. Hence, any patient who has pain in one leg after delivery should seek immediate medical attention.

Deep vein thrombosis is more common in the pregnant woman, owing to the effects of the hormone oestrogen, which makes the blood more likely to clot. It is also more likely to occur in patients who smoke, elderly patients or those who have undergone Caesarean section. Prolonged pressure on the leg veins by stirrups in the delivery position is another factor which predisposes the patient to deep vein thrombosis.

Examination of the patient is not enough for a proper diagnosis and special tests need to be done. One of these include ultrasound scans of the leg veins which would show blood flow to be affected over the blocked area. Another is a test called phlebography. In this test, a dye is injected into a vein on the surface of the foot. Television monitoring of the passage of the dye during injection would show up the area blocked by the clot.

Q How do we treat deep vein thrombosis?

A Drugs for dissolving blood clots (anticoagulants) such as heparin are used. After the initial period, maintenance of treatment is carried out over several weeks with another drug called coumarin to prevent a recurrence of the blood clot. If a large clot has travelled to the lungs, then an immediate operation to remove the clot (embolectomy) would be life-saving.

Q What are postnatal blues?

A This is a condition in which the patient becomes depressed, withdrawn, anxious and irritable after delivery. In severe cases, suicidal tendencies would surface. The usual patient who is suffering from postnatal depression is a first-time inexperienced mother with little family support. Contributory factors include pain from the breasts or episiotomy wound, fatigue, lack of sleep and a baby who cries without stopping. A previous episode of depression or mental problems is significant. The patient would usually behave in a slightly odd manner and get irritable over small issues. Instead of being happy at the arrival of the new baby, the patient keeps complaining about and reliving the unpleasant aspects of the whole labour process.

I had a telephone call from a patient at 3 a.m. one morning. She had had a normal delivery to a beautiful baby girl 2 weeks before and was physically very well. Her voice sounded very soft over the phone and she spoke with a slow, long drawl. Her husband was away on an urgent business trip and her mother-in-law was unsupportive towards her baby as she had wanted a grandson badly! My patient said that the baby had been crying non-stop for the past 6 hours, she was alone at home, her breasts hurt and the baby had just vomited. She asked me whether death would be instantaneous if she jumped off the eighth floor parapet with her baby!

It was fortunate that my nurse lived just in the next block of flats. After calling for the ambulance, I called my nurse and asked her to run over to the patient's apartment immediately. While waiting for the ambulance, my nurse kept chatting with the patient in the living room, cradling the baby all the time. The ambulance soon arrived and the patient was brought to hospital and given sedation. Her depression improved over the next few days with the return of her husband and improved family support.

In general, postnatal depression can be treated with minor tranquillizers. However, in some cases, especially those with previous episodes of severe depression, psychiatric help would be necessary.

Pointers for parenting

Chapter 2 addressed the issue of genetic endowment but an equally, if not more important, issue is that of nurture or the upbringing of a child.

Q How important is emotional bonding for the baby?

A The importance of the mother–child bond which occurs during the first few days of life is well-known. The continuing support of a nurturing family is vital for a child in all stages of his development. When social or emotional deprivation occurs and disrupts the early mutual bonding between baby and mother, psychological problems are bound to develop.

The normal child usually shows separation anxiety between 7 and 9 months of age. During this period, the child becomes anxious when his mother leaves his side or when others try to separate him from his mother. This clingy phase is an important step in the development of the mother-child bond. What this behaviour means is that the child has begun to realize he is a separate being and yet is dependant on his mother. After a few months he will realize her permanence and this anxiety will lessen.

The care and upbringing provided by the mother during the first 2 years should be reliable, consistent and warm, so that the child will develop a basic trust in the world around him. Indulgence is another matter. The child's experience of occasional frustrations and the appropriate delays in the fulfilment of his wishes would contribute to his social development and would further strengthen the mother-child relationship.

Mother-child bonding is but a part of the larger socialization process. The role of the father may be more variable as he is often the breadwinner and at work most of the day. However, fathers and siblings play an important function in stimulating the infant as well as in providing a 'secondary front' in the absence of the mother.

I am about to have another baby. How will this affect my present child?

 The birth of a new baby usually has a great impact on a child, who may respond in a variety of ways. This ranges from outright denial of the baby's birth to regressive actions like wetting or soiling his clothes and sucking his thumb. A child who is well-prepared will be able to accept the birth of the baby happily and hence the value of preparing the child psychologically for the arrival of the newborn. He must be reassured that he remains loved and even more so when baby actually comes.

He may have questions regarding how the baby came about and these questions should not be ignored. Instead, they should be answered factually, comfortably and with a good measure of love.

After the birth of our second child, we encouraged our older daughter to get really involved with his welfare such as changing his diapers and wiping his mouth after a feed. We never chided her on account of the baby boy as this would have sowed the seeds of animosity. We constantly heaped praises on her when praise was due.

How can we prevent the development of psychological problems in children?

The importance of spending quality time with your children cannot be over-emphasized. Sitting next to your child and watching television while he tries his utmost to tell you how his day went is not exactly spending quality time with him. Quality time means COMMUNICATION – wholesome, unrestrained, honest and consistent communication.

Consistency of communication is important because the parent who tells the child one thing in words while communicating the opposite in her actions will make the child confused. For example, in the presence of house guests, a noisy child may be told to go and play football in the garden for exercise. He will be confused because even though Mum says the exercise will be good for him, the frown on her face says something else. He probably can guess that she really wants him out of the way.

Being consistent in parenting extends into the area of discipline. Children who can predict what will happen if they behave badly are less likely to repeat such behaviour and are more likely to learn to take responsibility for their actions.

On the other hand, good deeds should be amply rewarded and appreciated to create positive reinforcement. Just as I was working on my notebook writing this chapter, my elder daughter came up with a piece of home-made chocolate cake – her first. I wolfed it down and asked for another piece. She squealed in genuine delight, gave me a big hug and ran off to get another piece. It may not have been the fanciest of cakes baked by a master chef but it was dripping with love and was arguably the most delicious cake that I have ever eaten.

Q My child is hyperactive. What do I do?

A The parents of a highly active child should realize that such a child needs a highly structured and consistent environment. Such a child will feel more secure when meal times, bedtimes and waking times are kept relatively constant and predictable from day to day. This pattern of basic security is a necessary foundation for the confidence he needs to cope with the unexpected events later in his life. In fact, this kind of orderly stable home environment is well-known to be conducive to the psychological well-being of children in general, but more so for the hyperactive child. A disorganized, unstable home where parents quarrel is the perfect setting for the development of psychological problems in children.

 How do we handle temper tantrums?

 Temper tantrums are common and usually peaks when a child is about 2 to $2^1/_2$ years of age. Parents should realize that these tantrums are used by the child to get attention and are also outward manifestations of his frustration at situations which he has no power to change. An example would be the crying fit when a child who is not sleepy is told to go to bed.

Provided parents stand their ground, the child soon learns that tantrums are useless and thereafter readily stops misbehaving as he realizes that it would get him nowhere.

What about anger in children?

Helping your child to cope with intense feelings can prevent serious psychological disorders from developing later on. For example, parents are advised to help a child verbalize his anger by asking the question, 'Why are you angry?' If no answer is forthcoming and if the parent knows the reason for the anger, then they can volunteer, 'You're angry because your brother ate up the cookie you were saving for tea, aren't you?' This often elicits a long verbal outburst and outpouring of the feelings of the offended child. A door has been opened to communication. The child will realize that anger is not wrong and it is good to have feelings, verbalize them and discuss them.

Learning to verbalize feelings and fears will stand the child in good stead for potentially stressful events in the future. These events could include the first day at school or even the first visit to the dentist. The parent should start by describing in clear, simple language what the child is about to go through. The child is then encouraged to express his feelings about the forthcoming event, be it fear or apprehension. Finally, the parent shows that he understands the child's feeling and at the same time corrects any misconception the child may have. This effectively defuses the stress that the child may otherwise feel.

Q My child refuses to go to school. What should I do?

A The refusal of a child to go to school is not uncommon in Nursery and Kindergarten. The children involved are usually good learners but tend to be somewhat fixed and spoilt in their ways. The parents should ensure that the child promptly returns to school. His continued attendance is also vital; otherwise a temporary refusal to go to school can develop into a long-standing problem.

We were somewhat unsympathetic to our son's reluctance to go to school until we discovered that there was a bully in class who was picking on him. A short chat with the teacher quickly solved the problem. (Not karate lessons.)

Q How far apart should we space our children?

A A gap of 2 to 3 years between siblings is felt to represent the optimal interval. From the medical point of view, the organs of reproduction would have returned to their pre-pregnancy state and any weakness or anaemia would have been corrected by good nutrition (please see the recipes earlier in this chapter) and exercise. From the social point of view, this spacing allows optimal mother-infant bonding to occur and by the time the next baby comes along, the older child would be starting to show the beginnings of his own independence and social development.

Q My children consistently fight. Is this normal?

A Bickering and competition among siblings are normal social responses and are important in the development of interpersonal skills necessary for survival in later life. Rough-and-tumble play is also important in the social development of the children as it establishes an hierarchy within the family. As long as this remains consistent, it forms a stable platform for growth and development. My son looks up to his older sister and tries to emulate her achievements.

Sometimes, however, arguments between siblings can become irrational and unhealthy, for example, when one child harbours malice or plots against the other. Parents who are in close contact with their children and who are in constant communication would quickly realize this and correct the situation with firm discipline and love.

How Many, How Soon?

There was an old woman who lived in a shoe,
She had so many children she did not know what to do.
So she fed them all cold broth without bread,
Spanked them soundly and sent them off to bed.

Poor woman. She probably had no means of contraception, natural or otherwise. But if she did, would she use them? And which method would she have picked? Many couples use a form of contraception not so much as to prevent pregnancies indefinitely but more as a means of planning when and how many children to have. Many methods are available and these are tabulated below :

Contraceptive methods and their relative effectiveness

Vaginal douching after intercourse	Not reliable
Withdrawal before ejaculation	Success depends very much on the couple being motivated, especially the husband
Rhythm/ Mucothermic	Approximately 60 to 85% safe and depends very much on the fertility of the couple
Spermicides	Unreliable when used on its own. Occasionally produces an itch in the woman.
Condom/Cap	Fairly safe if used correctly

Progesterone-only pill	Failure rate of about 2 to 4%
Intrauterine contraceptive device	Good in that success is independent of user. Failure rate of 2 to 3%
Family planning pill (Combined pill)	Very effective and reliable if the woman does not forget and takes the pill according to the instructions. Failure rates of only 0.1 to 0.3%
Levonorgestrel implant	Highly effective. Not dependant on the user. Failure rate of 0.1 to 0.2%
'Morning after' contraception	This is for emergency use only, e.g. after a burst condom. Failure rate of 1%
Sterilization/ Vasectomy	Very effective, with failure rates of less than 0.2% if done properly. The main disadvantage is the permanence of the method in the event that the couple wishes to have children in future.

Douching

Q What is douching?

A Douching is the washing of the vagina with a cleansing solution. This is done some time after sexual intercourse, with the hope that it would remove the sperms and prevent fertilization. Numerous preparations, ranging from a solution of baking powder to Coca Cola, have been used but douching is usually ineffective in preventing pregnancies. This is because immediately after ejaculation, many sperms would have found their way into the neck of the womb. There they would be protected by the mucus in the cervix.

Withdrawal method

Q What is the withdrawal method? How safe is it for family planning?

A In the withdrawal method, unprotected sexual intercourse is practised but the husband withdraws just before ejaculation, which takes place outside the vagina. This method may fail because of premature ejaculation. Also, secretions from the penis before ejaculation (the pre-ejaculate) occasionally contain enough sperms to fertilize a woman if she is highly fertile.

Q What do you mean by a highly fertile woman?

A A woman is presumed to be highly fertile if she is between the ages of 18 to 33 years or if she is within the fertile period of her menstrual cycle. This extends from day 9 to day 19 of a normal 28-day menstrual cycle. A woman is of lower fertility when she is breast feeding. However, fertilization and pregnancy can still occur during this period.

Rhythm method

Q What is the rhythm method?

A The essence of this method is to predict the exact time of ovulation and to have unprotected sexual intercourse outside this time. This is the method acceptable to Catholics. The rhythm method is useful only in women who have very regular menstrual cycles. Ovulation usually takes place 14 days before the onset of the menstruation. That is to say, ovulation takes place on day 14 of a 28-day cycle, day 16 of a 30-day cycle or day 19 of a 33-day cycle. In a normal menstrual cycle, the first half, from onset of menstruation to ovulation, is variable whereas the second half, from ovulation to the start of the next cycle, is constant.

The difficulties inherent in this method are obvious. The exact time of ovulation may vary from cycle to cycle in the same woman. Also, the time of ovulation can only be known RETROSPECTIVELY, when the menses starts. As such, the ease with which 'accidents' can arise is clear.

The reliability of the rhythm method can be increased by using an ovulation predictor. A urine sample is taken at the time of ovulation and a change in colour of the test kit indicates ovulation and therefore high fertility. However, these over-the-counter kits are not always dependable.

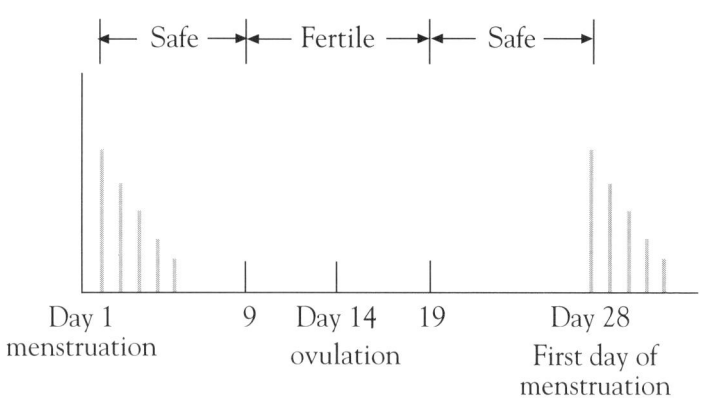

A 28-day menstrual cycle

Q   Why is the mucothermic method thus named?

A   This comes from two words – 'mucus' and 'thermal'. At the time of ovulation, the mucus discharge from the vagina is clear and stringy, like egg white. If a sample is held between forefinger and thumb, it can be stretched until a bridge of 10 cm is formed without the mucus breaking. This indicates ovulation and therefore high fertility. If the temperature is recorded daily using a special ovulation thermometer, the time of ovulation can be detected by a slight fall and then a sustained rise in temperature of 0.3 to 0.5°C. The dip and rise again reflects ovulation and therefore high fertility. Unprotected intercourse is therefore avoided before and for 4 days after the rise in temperature. Failures can occur because ovulation can sometimes occur without these changes in cervical mucus or temperature. Also, sperms can live for many days in the cervix of the woman so that fertilization can occur even many days after sexual intercourse.

Q Why are spermicides ineffective when used alone?

A Spermicides are chemicals which kill sperms. Pessaries, sponges impregnated with spermicides, creams, pastes, or foaming tablets are sometimes inserted into the vagina as a form of contraceptive. A man must truly be in love to have sexual intercourse with a woman foaming in the vagina! This is not usually effective when used alone. Imagine trying to kill 200 million little sperms. Some are bound to get away! Spermicides are more effective when combined with another method like a barrier method.

Barrier methods

Q What are barrier methods of family planning?

A These are the condom or French cap for the man and the diaphragm or Dutch cap for the woman. (One wonders in the naming of these devices whether the British had a bone to pick with their neighbours!) Both the condom and diaphragm act by preventing the sperms from entering the womb and meeting the egg. Hence, the term 'barrier' method.

Q What is a condom?

A The basic model is a thin rubber sheath which looks like an elongated balloon with a little nipple at its tip to contain semen. More advanced devices include ribbed condoms to enhance sensation for the woman, as well as coloured condoms.

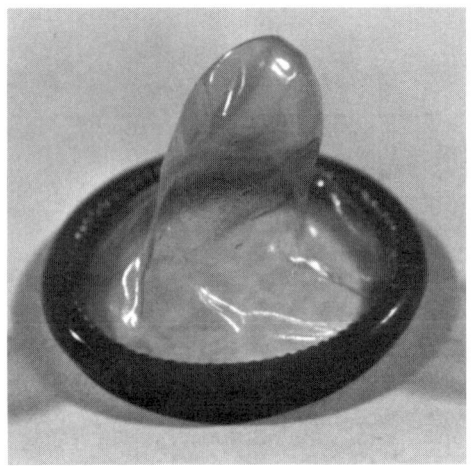

A condom

Q What are the advantages and disadvantages of using the condom?

A The condom is easily available in supermarkets and 7-eleven stores. Its main advantage is that it is easily used and has no side-effects. More importantly, it protects the user from a variety of sexually transmitted diseases.

The disadvantage of the condom is that many men hate to use it as it decreases sensation. It also destroys the spontaneity of the sex act. Some women who are allergic to rubber may complain of an itch.

 How is a condom used?

 A condom should be rolled onto the penis up to the base before any genital contact. A little space is left at the top to collect semen after ejaculation. Following intercourse, the penis should be withdrawn while still erect, with the man or woman holding on to the rim of the rubber sheath at the base of the penis. This is to prevent the condom from being left behind in the vagina as the penile erection subsides.

There is this story of a man whose wife became pregnant even though he used the condom. 'I don't understand it. I rolled the condom onto my left thumb every time we had sex, just like they did at the family planning talk. It just didn't work!'

 What is a diaphragm?

 This is a rubber device shaped like a shallow cap. It has a wire around its edge to help it keep its shape and to ensure that it stays in place when used. Diaphragms come in various sizes ranging from 60 mm to 100 mm in diameter.

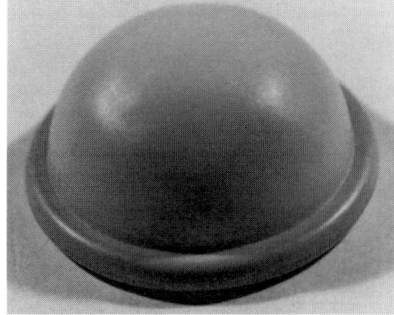

A diaphragm

Q   What are the advantages and disadvantages of using a diaphragm?

A   The advantages of using a diaphragm are that it need not be inserted and removed during sexual excitement, and that it is managed by the woman, who has an infinitely greater interest that pregnancy does not happen than the man. The disadvantage is that the diaphragm has to be fitted for the correct size by a trained gynaecologist prior to usage and this fit must be checked after 1 week, 2 months and then annually if all goes well. Pregnancy, increasing sexual activity, changes in weight and body fat and increasing age are factors which may require the diaphragm to be refitted. Diaphragm users may develop itchiness due to sensitivity to the rubber. They also have an increased incidence of urinary tract infection.

Q   How exactly is a diaphragm used?

A   After applying a spermicide to both surfaces of the device, the woman is taught how to place the diaphragm into the vagina so as to completely cover the neck of the womb. She does this by standing with one leg on a low chair, squeezing the diaphragm between thumb and forefinger and sliding it into the vagina. The rim of the diaphragm is then felt to ensure that the cervix is covered. After sexual intercourse, the diaphragm is left in place for at least 6 hours before it is removed. With repeated intercourse, more spermicide should be inserted into the vagina without dislodging the diaphragm.

The diaphragm deteriorates with time. Hence all these devices should be checked by the woman at regular intervals for defects in the rubber, and changed if necessary. After a period of 2 years, all diaphragms should be changed. Good motivation is essential for diaphragm or condom usage to be successful. Couples who find its use troublesome should employ other methods of contraception.

The intrauterine contraceptive device (IUCD)

Q What is an intrauterine contraceptive device (IUCD)?

A This is an interesting form of family planning with a unique history. Camels were the mainstay of transport along the old silk route, carrying goods from China across northern Asia to the Middle East. Often, the bedouins would tear their hair out in desperation as these camels would become pregnant, making them unfit to carry their precious loads of silk and spices. Then one day, a desperate (or frustrated) trader put a small stone into the womb of a camel. Lo and behold, this was the only camel that did not become pregnant on the long and arduous journey. This practice quickly caught on and what is good for the camel must be good for the human. Hence the intrauterine contraceptive device (IUCD) was born. Of course we do not use rocks or pebbles. Instead we use pretty little soft plastic devices with copper wires wound around them to increase their effectiveness.

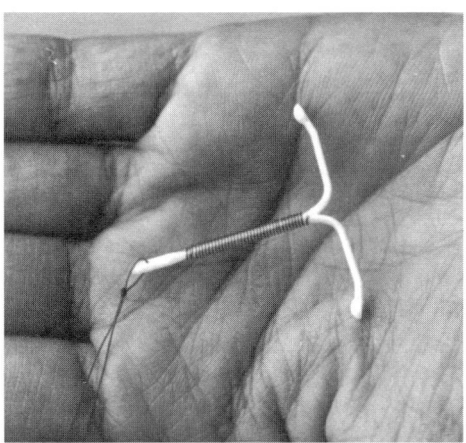

An intrauterine contraceptive device (IUCD)

How does the IUCD work?

 It affects the movement of the egg within the Fallopian tube so that the critical timing required for the egg to meet the sperm is disrupted. Also, the copper affects the action of the enzymes necessary for the attachment of the embryo to the wall of the womb.

 Who are the patients who use the IUCD?

The IUCD is useful for women who find other methods unacceptable. It is useful for breast feeding women, older women or for those who see their husbands occasionally. In particular, the IUCD is well-suited for the woman who wants a fuss-free method – once it is inserted, the woman herself needs to do nothing more. The IUCD is also a useful alternative for patients who are unable to take the pill for medical reasons.

 Are there any side-effects when using the IUCD?

The most frequent problems with IUCD use are heavy menstrual bleeding and low abdominal pains, usually during the menses in the first few months after insertion of the device. Rarely does it lead to infection of the tissues around the womb (pelvic inflammatory disease) or an ectopic pregnancy.

Who cannot use an IUCD?

The IUCD should not be used by women with heavy menstruation, those with abnormal wombs, women who have had pelvic infections before or those who are on steroid therapy, as this increases the risk of serious infections occurring. Vaginal infections, if any, should be treated before an IUCD is inserted.

Q How is an IUCD inserted? Is it painful?

A An IUCD is inserted by a trained doctor in a proper clinic. This is because a strictly sterile field is essential to decrease the incidence of pelvic infections. It is done during the first half of the menstrual cycle to avoid inserting the IUCD in a womb with a fetus. With the patient lying on her back and her legs suspended by stirrups, a metal speculum is inserted. The neck of the womb is then held by a pair of forceps (a device like a thin pair of tongs) and the plastic IUCD inserted with the help of a plastic introducer. The only slight discomfort is felt when the cervix is held and the device inserted. The whole procedure takes only a minute. The patient is then taught how to put her finger into the vagina to feel for the IUCD thread and confirm that it is in place. Only rarely is an injection of local anaesthesia needed for an IUCD insertion.

Q Is any after-care needed?

A The IUCD should be checked a month after insertion by the doctor because it occasionally gets out of position (translocated). Having established that the IUCD is in the correct position in the womb, periodic examinations are advised to monitor the extent of menstrual bleeding and to check for infection in the vagina.

How long can an IUCD last?

This depends on the particular device. The average span of time is $2^1/_2$ years, after which the IUCD should be removed and changed, or some other method used. Newer devices have a longer life span of up to 5 years but there is a marginally increased risk of pelvic infection.

How is an IUCD removed?

This is usually a simple and painless procedure done in the doctor's clinic without any anaesthesia. After inserting a speculum into the vagina, the IUCD thread is located and gently pulled. The IUCD follows the thread and is thereby removed. Only in rare cases can the thread not be seen. Removal of the IUCD is then tricky and a D & C may be required for its removal.

Drugs

What form of family planning involves the use of drugs?

Drugs used for family planning are essentially hormones and can be given in three forms: the oral or combined pill, the progesterone-only pill and injections of progesterone either once every 2 months, or by inserting tubes of the hormone levonorgestrel under the skin.

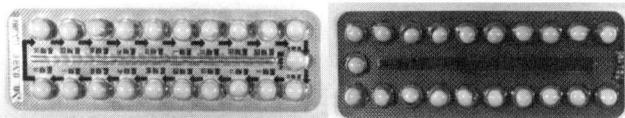

Combined pills for contraception

Q What is the combined pill?

A The combined pill is a commonly used form of contraception. Each pill contains the two main female hormones oestrogen and progesterone in artificial form. There are many different brands but essentially each pack has 21 pills which are used over 1 month.

Q How is the pill taken?

A Each packet of the combined pill contains 21 tablets and are numbered according to the days of the week. Beginning from the 3rd day of the menstrual cycle, one pill is swallowed every morning at the same time each day. After 3 weeks, the last pill in the packet would have been consumed. After a few more days, the menses would appear and this is usually of a lighter flow than normal. A week after the last pill was taken, a new pack of pills would be started. That is to say, if the first pill of the pack was taken on a Monday, then the last pill would be taken 3 weeks later on a Sunday. The next pack would then be started again on a Monday a week later. Numbering the pills according to the days of the week helps the patient to check whether she has forgotten to take the pill on any particular day.

Q How does the pill work?

A The pill acts by preventing the release of the egg. It also affects the lining of the womb so that it becomes unsuitable for attachment of an embryo. The pill also prevents pregnancy by making the mucus of the neck of the womb thick, so that sperms have trouble swimming through it.

Q   Are there any serious side-effects when taking the pill?

A   Serious side-effects with pill usage are rare. The main side-effects are associated with blood clotting problems. These include clotting of blood in the veins of the legs (deep vein thrombosis), blocking of main blood vessels in the lungs by a blood clot (pulmonary embolism), heart attacks (myocardial infarction) and strokes (cerebral thrombosis). The risks of these major side-effects occurring are markedly increased in obese patients above the age of 35, in smokers, and in patients with diabetes, high blood pressure and high blood cholesterol levels. Other side-effects include depression, migraine, worsening of mild diabetes or epileptic fits and non-cancerous growths of the liver.

Q   What are the less serious side-effects of pill usage?

A   These include slight irregular bleeding while taking the pill (breakthrough bleeding), failure to menstruate on stopping use of the pill, weight gain, dryness of the vagina and a diminished sex drive.

The less common side-effects are a slight increase in facial hair or pimples, anxiety or mild depression, nausea, darkening of the skin of the face (chloasma) and a feeling of bloatedness in the abdomen.

Q   What are the beneficial effects of pill use?

A   Besides preventing unwanted pregnancies, the pill decreases menstrual blood loss and hence is very useful in patients with heavy menses. Pill usage also decreases the risk of cancer of the womb and ovary. Rheumatoid arthritis and thyroid disease as well as premenstrual tension improves with pill use.

Q Who cannot take the pill?

A The oral contraceptive pill should not be used by patients who have had heart disease or blood clotting problems before, those who have had cancer of the breast or womb, those with diabetes, high blood pressure, high blood cholesterol levels, chronic liver infections and mood problems. The pill is also unsuitable for breast feeding mothers as the milk flow would decrease with pill usage.

Q Are there different types of pills for different women?

A Basically, the pill used should contain the lowest possible level of the hormones oestrogen and progesterone effective for birth control. Women with menstrual problems should be given a pill with a higher progesterone component. However, those who have mild depression, weight gain or dryness of the vagina should have a pill with a lower progesterone or higher oestrogen content. Sometimes, a patient suffers headaches while she is on the pill. In such a case, changing either component in turn with different formulations would be necessary to find a brand which does not cause this problem.

Q Can I take any other medication when I am on the pill?

A The pill does interfere with the action of certain other drugs. It reduces the effect of drugs for diabetes and high blood pressure. Hence the dosage for these drugs may need to be increased. On the other hand, the effects of steroids which are given for diseases like asthma or skin diseases are more pronounced and the dosage will need to be decreased. Certain drugs also reduce the effectiveness of the pill. These include antibiotics like ampicillin and tetracyclines, drugs which control fits, and medication used in the treatment of tuberculosis (TB). When on these medications, the contraceptive pill has lowered effectiveness and some other form of family planning may need to be used.

Q Is there a contraceptive pill which can be used in breast-feeding women?

A The progesterone-only pill is suitable for breast feeding women. In this form, the dose of progesterone is lower than that found in the combined pill. As such, the side-effects encountered with the combined pill are much less. The progesterone-only pill also increases the production of breast milk. However, the contraceptive effectiveness is lower than that of the combined pill and hence the progesterone-only pill is suitable for women with lowered fertility. These include breast feeding women and those above the age of 40 years.

The progesterone-only pill is also prescribed for women with diabetes, high blood pressure or those with a previous experience of blood clotting problems as these women are unable to take the combined pill.

Q Is there any side-effect with the progesterone-only pill?

A The only side-effect which is troublesome is disturbance of menstruation. This includes irregular spotting and heavy bleeding, which may occur even after many months of use. If patients with bleeding problems persist with the progesterone-only pill, such bleeding usually settles down to a more acceptable pattern.

Q How is the progesterone-only pill taken?

A This pill is taken once a day at the same time each day. It is also very important that the progesterone-only pill is taken several hours before sexual intercourse for increased efficacy.

Q What are injectable progestogens?

A These are progesterone compounds which are given in the form of injections once every 2 to 3 months.

Q What are the advantages of injectable progestogens?

A The advantages of injectable progestogens are that they are effective, convenient and easy to give. They do not decrease breast milk production, free the patient from having to remember to swallow pills daily and are also devoid of such side-effects of the hormone oestrogen as blood clotting problems.

Q Are there any disadvantages to this form of family planning?

A The major disadvantage is that once given, none of the effects of the drug can be reversed for the duration of activity of the drug. This may last up to 5 months. Other disadvantages are a disturbance in menstruation, no menstruation after one year of use (in 30 per cent of patients), very heavy menstruation with some requiring a D & C, and a slight increase in weight. However, in most women, normal menstrual cycles resume after 6 months following the last injection and fertility is not affected.

Q   What is the levonorgestrel implant?

A   This is a form of injectable progesterone which has the advantage of being as effective as the combined pill, without the side-effects of oestrogens. The beauty of this method is that after the insertion, the contraceptive effect lasts for 5 years.

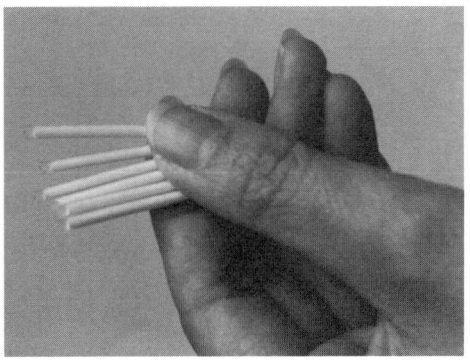

Levonogestrel implants

Q   How is the levonorgestrel implant inserted?

A   This is inserted into the inner side of the arm just above the elbow. The patient lies on a couch and the inner side of the left arm is cleaned with iodine solution to kill the surface bacteria. A local anaesthetic is then given and a small cut made in the skin. Using a metal tube, six little plastic tubes are pushed under the skin in a fan-shaped pattern. A plaster is put over the surface wound and the arm bandaged. There will be some surface bruising but this clears after a week. Once in place, the levonorgestrel implant can be felt under the skin but cannot be seen. Also, its presence does not affect arm movements in any way and all forms of physical activity, e.g. swimming, are possible.

Q What are the side-effects of the levenorgestrel implant?

A This is mainly disturbance of menstruation, e.g. irregular bleeding and absence of menstruation. These problems, although distressing, are usually temporary. Irregular bleeding can be temporarily arrested with a short course of the combined pill.

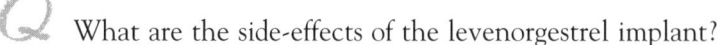

Stopping for good

Q What permanent methods are there for preventing pregnancies?

A These are sterilization procedures which can be performed either on the woman or the man. Before advising such a procedure, I usually take into consideration the age of both husband and wife, the number and ages of their children, their economic background and the stability of their marriage. It is important that both partners understand fully the nature of the procedure and that no method is 100 per cent safe although failure rates are extremely low.

Q How is sterilization (ligation) of the woman performed?

A This is done as an operation either immediately after the birth of the baby, at the time of a Caesarean section or as an interval procedure, that is, many months or years after delivery.

If done immediately after delivery, a 1-cm cut is made just below the navel to locate the Fallopian tubes. At the time of Caesarean section, no additional incision is necessary and ligation is performed through the same cut. If done as an interval procedure, ligation is usually performed under laparoscopy and the patient can return home the very same day. In all methods, the ligation is done with the patient under general anaesthesia (or epidural in the case of a Caesarean section) and the tubes cut and a portion removed, burned or clipped to block the hole. This prevents the egg from travelling through the tube to meet the sperm.

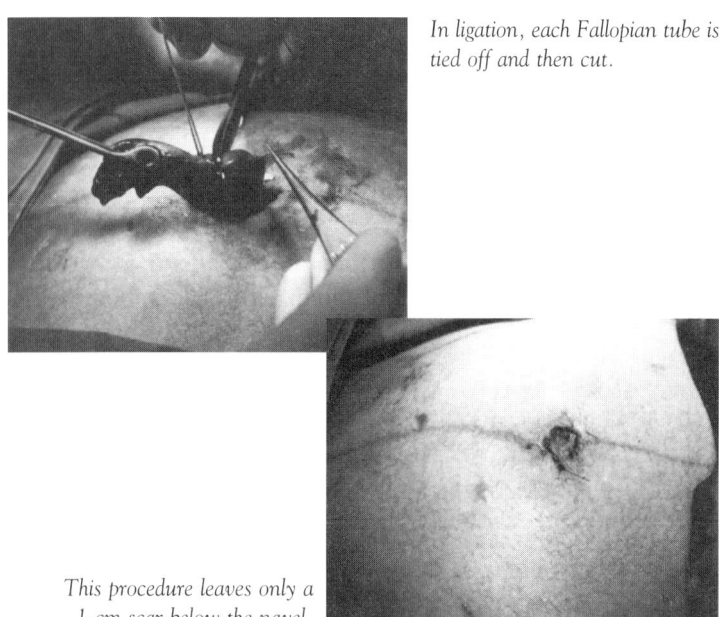

In ligation, each Fallopian tube is tied off and then cut.

This procedure leaves only a 1-cm scar below the navel.

Q Will ligation cause a woman to put on weight? Are there any side-effects?

A Ligation of a woman's Fallopian tubes will not cause her to put on more weight and has no ill effects on her general health whatsoever. This is because there is no change in hormone production as the ovaries are not involved. A mild, low abdominal pain may be present for a short while but this soon settles after a week.

Q Is this procedure reversible?

A How successful the reversal of a ligation process is depends on the amount of Fallopian tube destroyed and the length of time since the operation. In general, a 70 per cent success rate can be achieved but the reversal process involves a complicated operation in which the tubes are rejoined with the help of an operating microscope.

Q What is a vasectomy?

A A vasectomy is an operation to sterilize the man. This is a relatively simple procedure and is performed as an outpatient procedure under local anaesthesia. Two small cuts are made high in the scrotum. The vas deferens is identified and a portion removed. This prevents the sperms produced in the testes from reaching the urethra. Hence the ejaculate is devoid of sperms.

Q What are the possible complications?

A A blood clot may form at the operation site, causing pain and even infection. Bruising and pain for a week after the procedure is common and usually medical leave for a few days is necessary. Also, unlike ligation in the female, a vasectomy is not immediately effective. As there are sperms stored beyond the level where the cut is made, the partner must use some other form of family planning for a few months until no more sperms are seen in the semen under microscopic examination.

Q   Can a vasectomy be reversed?

A   This is possible but even though sperms can be seen in the ejaculate in 65 per cent of patients after the cut ends of the vas deferens are rejoined, only half of these would result in a successful pregnancy.

When accidents happen ...

Q   Help! We could not find the condom after intercourse!

A   This is not uncommon. Withdrawal of the penis after it has become flaccid can result in the condom being left behind in the vagina. As there is a 20 to 30 per cent risk of pregnancy especially if you are in the fertile part of the cycle, postcoital contraception will be needed.

Q   What is postcoital contraception?

A   Postcoital contraception is used to prevent pregnancy following unprotected intercourse. This should be given as soon as possible after the episode and comprises two possible methods: hormones and the IUCD.

Q   How can hormones be used for postcoital contraception?

A   Two tablets of the combined pill are given immediately after the patient is seen and another two 12 hours later. This is a special pill containing 50 micrograms of ethinyl-oestradiol and 250 micrograms of levonorgestrel. Side-effects are nausea and vomiting and this can be controlled with anti-nausea tablets.

Q What if the patient cannot tolerate the combined pill?

A Then the IUCD is inserted as soon as possible. This does not cause nausea and vomiting but some patients complain of discomfort at the time of insertion and pain and bleeding a few days later.

10 Sexually Transmitted Diseases (STDs) – Don'ts and More Don'ts

The husband of a patient of mine, a father of four lovely children, recently went on a business trip abroad. On the way home en route to the airport, in a moment of rare abandon, he spent just 10 minutes in a brothel. Two weeks later, full of remorse and sick as a dog, he came to my clinic with a combination of herpes, gonorrhoea and pubic lice. He is at present waiting in anguish as the HIV test may not show positive until 6 months later.

As for most illnesses, a changing pattern is apparent in the occurrence of sexually transmitted diseases (STDs). In the sixties, we saw the spread of the hippie movement. Sympathizers called the hippies 'saintly wanderers, living in self-imposed exile, in search of their ideals'. Many hippies unfortunately not only left their homes, they also left their morals behind and advocated free love. Syphilis then spread like wildfire through the communes and beyond.

Then in the seventies, there was the Vietnam War. Young men were thrown into a conflict many did not believe in, shot at enemies they did not hate and spent nights in brothels trying to forget the anguish of a war they did not understand. Gonorrhoea became rampant and the emergence of drug-resistant forms was a major health concern for the military. Unfortunately, infected servicemen then carried the disease home and gonorrhoea became the scourge of many urban cities.

In the eighties, many men and women started complaining of pain on passing urine and yet tests performed on the urine yielded no bacteria. Later, specific tests revealed the culprit to be an evasive little bug called *Chlamydia*.

Now, we are in the nineties and the latest STDs are the human papillomavirus (HPV) and the fearsome HIV or AIDS virus.

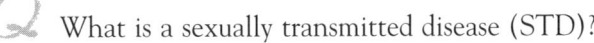

Sexually transmitted diseases (STDs)

Q   What is a sexually transmitted disease (STD)?

A   A sexually transmitted disease is a disease which is primarily transmitted through sexual activity. The organism which causes it could be a bacteria (against which antibiotics would work) or a virus (against which antibiotics are useless). It could also be something in between, like the mycoplasma, against which some antibiotics work.

Q   What are the warning signs of an STD?

A   There are ten common symptoms of STDs in the woman:

1. Increased amount of discharge from the vagina. The colour may be yellow, green, blood-stained or have a foul smell
2. Blisters or sores of any kind in the genital area
3. Itching around the entrance of the vagina, anus or where the pubic hair is
4. Pain during intercourse, usually at the entrance of the vagina or deeper low abdominal pain
5. Pain with a burning sensation when passing urine or passing motion

6. Pain in the lower abdomen or back. This is typically worse on deep pressure or during coughing or sneezing
7. Unusually severe low abdominal pain during menstruation
8. Vaginal bleeding after sexual intercourse
9. Fever with shivering
10. Unexplained tiredness

What are the common STDs in women?

These can be divided into diseases that frequently produce early symptoms and those in which symptoms appear late.

STDs with early symptoms

Disease	Caused by
Vaginitis	*Candida albicans* *Trichomonas vaginalis*
Genital herpes	*Herpes simplex* virus type 2
Gonorrhoea	*Neisseria gonococcus*
Non-specific urethritis (NSU)	*Chlamydia*
Syphilis	*Treponema pallidum*
Chancroid	*Haemophilus ducreyi*
Lymphogranuloma venereum	*Chlamydia trachomatis*
Granuloma inguinale	*Calymmatobacterium granulomatis*
Molluscum contagiosum	Poxvirus
Genital warts (condyloma acuminata)	Human papillomavirus (HPV)

STDs with delayed symptoms

Disease	Caused by
Precancerous change of the cervix, vagina and vulva	Human papillomavirus (HPV)
Acquired immune deficiency syndrome (AIDS)	Human immunodeficiency virus (HIV)

Vaginitis and cervicitis

Q What is vaginitis? What causes it?

A Vaginitis is infection of the vagina and the two commonest organisms causing it are the fungus *Candida albicans* and the parasite *Trichomonas vaginalis*. While *Candida* infection is not an STD *per se*, it can be passed from woman to man. *Trichomonas* infection, on the other hand, is an STD.

Q What are the symptoms of vaginitis?

A Vaginitis causes an increased discharge and itching of the skin around the lower vagina. *Candida* typically produces a cheesy thick white discharge with no smell and the itchiness is worse after the menses. *Trichomonas*, on the other hand, produces a frothy, fishy-smelling, greyish-green discharge with itchiness that is worse during the menses. Both organisms can be identified through a simple microscopic examination of a sample of the vaginal discharge.

Q How is vaginitis treated?

A *Candida* infection is treated using pessaries of an anti-fungal agent and *Trichomonas* infection with a drug called metronidazole. For *Candida*, an anti-fungus drug taken orally would reduce the rate of future infections as the *Candida* spores are found in the intestines and these spores can infect the vagina if left untreated.

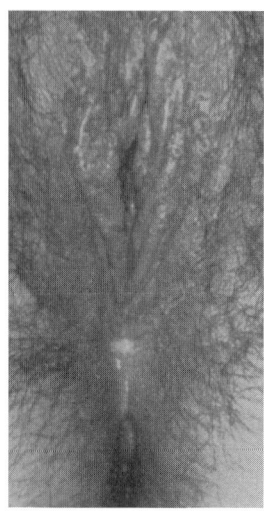

Vaginitis caused by Candida albicans

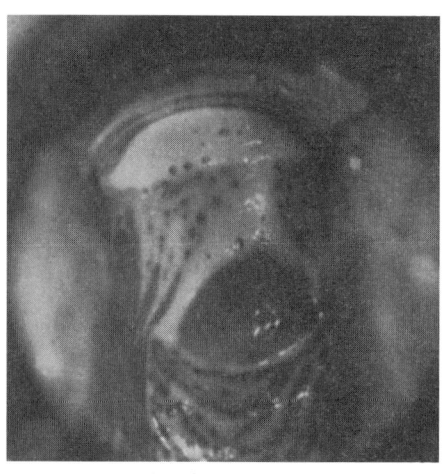

A cervix infected with Candida albicans as seen through a speculum

What is cervicitis?

Cervicitis is infection of the neck of the womb (cervix) and this occurs in two forms:

1. Endocervicitis, the commoner condition, is an infection of the canal of the neck of the womb. This is usually caused by *Neisseria gonorrhoea* or *Chlamydia trachomatis*.

2. Ectocervicitis, which is an infection of the outer portion of the neck of the womb, is usually caused by the *Herpes simplex* virus or the human papillomavirus.

Q How is cervicitis treated?

A Cervicitis is treated after first identifying the organism causing the infection. For *Neisseria gonorrhoea* and *Chlamydia trachomatis*, the treatment is with penicillins, tetracyclines or spectinomycin. Infection with HSV or HPV will not respond to antibiotics as these are viruses. The infection can only be eradicated by methods which destroy the infected cells and this can be done using laser vaporization, freezing (cryosurgery) or burning (electrocautery or diathermy).

Herpes

Q What is herpes?

A Herpes is an infection caused by the *Herpes simplex* virus of which there are two types. *Herpes simplex* type 1 causes ulcers around the mouth and *Herpes simplex* type 2 causes infections around the genital area. It is mainly the latter that is significant in STDs.

Q How long after sexual contact will the herpes infection appear?

A After exposure to the *Herpes* virus, there will usually be an incubation period of 2 to 7 days before the symptoms appear.

Q What are the symptoms of genital herpes?

A Infection around the entrance of the vagina is seen as painful fluid-filled blisters. The surrounding skin appears red and inflamed. Sometimes, a vaginal discharge is present. The patient is likely to have a fever with tiredness, headaches, muscle pains, nausea and pain on passing urine. The lymph nodes of the groin are also usually painful and swollen. The blisters usually appear at the opening to the vagina (vulva), buttocks, neck of the womb (cervix) and vagina. The blisters soon break down to form painful shallow ulcers and these may last for 12 to 20 days. A first-person account of a *herpes* victim follows:

My world was shattered one night after dinner. We had put the children to bed when my husband broke down. He had caught herpes from a girl he had met at a karaoke lounge. I felt an icy hand grip my heart. I felt like killing him – bringing germs from some slut into my home! I took a long, hard look at myself. I am 37 years old, pretty and vivacious. I hung on to my self-esteem. I told myself never to let a man's weakness and a slut destroy me. But what made him do it, I wondered over and over again.

It was my training as an accountant that saved me. I was taught to be logical. First things first. I knew I was at risk because we did not use the condom during intercourse. I steeled myself for the first signs of infection. Ten days after the fateful confession, it happened.

It started as a warm feeling on passing urine. A cold chill ran through me and I looked at my vagina with a mirror. There was nothing. The next morning, my head felt like exploding. I felt nauseous and my vagina felt as though it was on fire. I could not even part my legs or take normal strides.

My gynaecologist confirmed it was herpes. On the TV screen above, I could see many small blisters all over the entrance of my vagina. He was very comforting and he cleansed my vagina with a soothing liquid. He then prescribed some tablets to prevent the spread of the Herpes virus. The next day, I was slightly better but passing urine was still sheer torture. I suffered terribly for the next few days. I ran a temperature and my whole body ached. My vagina still felt very sore and I had to cleanse it with a yellow solution called acriflavine to prevent further infection.

Only after a week did I feel much better and was able to go about normally. It was difficult to contemplate suicide with two lovely girls at home. The only reason that I was persuaded to write about my private, hellish experience is that I want all husbands and wives who are contemplating extra-marital affairs to have a glimpse of the physical agony and the mental anguish it can cause. My husband has been extremely remorseful and I have decided, for the sake of the children, to give him another chance.

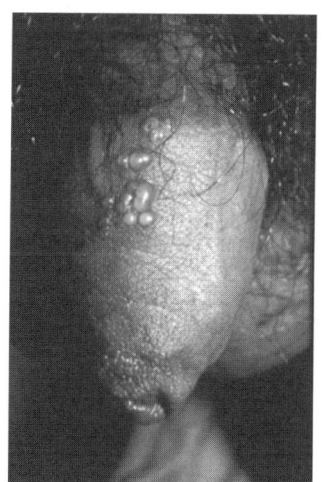

Herpes of the penis

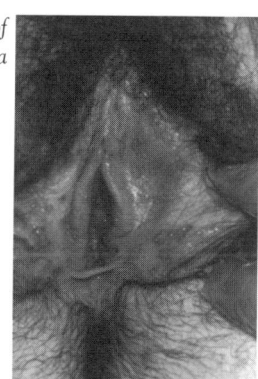

Herpes of the vulva

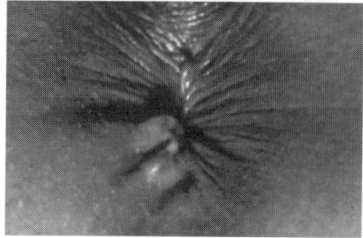

Herpes of the anus

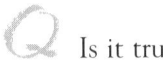 Is it true that herpes is a recurrent disease?

It has been said that for the woman, besides diamonds, herpes is also forever. Flare-ups of old herpes infections can occur. However, in recurrent infections, the extent of the blisters and ulcers is much less and general symptoms like fever and muscle aches are absent. A hard crust usually forms over the blisters within 4 days. The blisters then dry up and healing is usually complete within 10 days. Recurrent infections are usually heralded by a feeling of itchiness, tingling, nerve pains and a burning sensation over the genital area. After a few hours (or sometimes 1 or 2 days), the characteristic blisters of herpes appear. The rate of recurrence varies from person to person. It can be as often as every 2 to 3 weeks initially, to once every few months. Approximately half of the patients with genital herpes suffer from one or more recurrent attacks monthly.

 What brings on flare-ups of the old disease?

Flare-ups of old herpes infections occur especially when the resistance of the woman decreases, e.g. during pregnancy or menstruation, when under emotional stress, when undergoing steroid treatment and when suffering from a viral fever or an infection with another form of STD.

 How is genital herpes treated?

Effective treatment for genital infection with the *Herpes simplex* virus is now available in the form of acyclovir. This drug markedly shortens the duration of infection and reduces the incidence of recurrent infection. However, there is still no total cure for herpes infection as neither acyclovir nor any other agent is effective against latent viruses in the body.

Acyclovir in tablet form is the preferred medication for initial infections and this shortens the average length of initial infections by 4 to 6 days. It also lessens the intensity of the symptoms.

Acyclovir can also be given intravenously via an injection. This has also been found to be effective in decreasing the amount of viruses released by the blisters (and hence infectivity) and in reducing local and general symptoms like nausea and fever.

Q How soon should treatment be given for the initial infection?

A Treatment must begin within 6 days of the start of the blisters and continue for 10 days.

Q What about recurrent herpes?

A Continuous treatment with oral acyclovir is used to treat recurrent herpes. This is effective in reducing the number of recurrences by 60 to 80 per cent among patients with frequent recurrent attacks. Long-term treatment with acyclovir has been shown to be safe and effective for up to 2 years. This form of treatment also prolongs the interval between the end of a course of treatment and any subsequent recurrence.

Q Is the dosage of acyclovir the same for recurrent herpes?

A The treatment lasts for 5 days but must be given at the start of warning signs like skin tingling or within 2 days of appearance of blisters.

Gonorrhoea

Q What is gonorrhoea?

A Gonorrhoea is an STD caused by a bacteria known as *Neisseria gonorrhoea*. The initial site of the infection is usually the neck of the womb (cervix), the outer part of the urinary passage (urethra) and a gland at the lower part of the vagina (Bartholin's gland). The infection spreads quickly from the neck of the womb up through the body of the womb to the Fallopian tubes, which become swollen and inflamed. Pus may escape out of the Fallopian tubes to infect the tissues surrounding the womb (peritonitis or pelvic cellulitis).

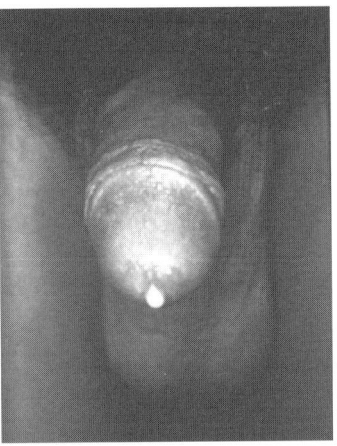

Gonorrhoea of the penis

Q What are the common symptoms of gonorrhoea infection?

A The patient complains of vaginal discharge and pain on passing urine a few days to a week after sexual contact with an infected partner. A low abdominal pain with tenderness and associated fever, nausea and vomiting is frequently present.

Q How can the diagnosis be confirmed?

A Apart from the above symptoms, an internal examination by the gynaecologist would reveal a sharp low abdominal pain when the neck of the womb is moved. The discharge from the urinary passage is sent to the laboratory, where examination under a microscope will reveal numerous white blood cells containing pairs of the characteristic round bacteria.

Q How is gonorrhoea treated?

A Uncomplicated gonorrhoea is treated using penicillin either orally or through intramuscular injections. Often, gonorrhoea exists together with another infection such as *Chlamydia* infection of the urinary passage. The antibiotic chosen must then be also effective against *Chlamydia* and a tetracycline compound may need to be used in this instance. Not uncommonly, one encounters strains of gonorrhoea which do not respond to penicillin treatment. For these cases, a more powerful drug called spectinomycin is used.

Q What else should a person with gonorrhoea do?

A The patient should identify the source of her infection so that he can be treated. Sex must be avoided until the patient and her partner are both cured. Thereafter, condoms should be used to prevent future infections. She should understand when and how to take her medication and do it faithfully so that a cure can be achieved. She should also see her gynaecologist a week after completing treatment so that tests can be done to confirm she is cured. She should also return early if the pain on passing urine or vaginal discharge persists or recurs.

Non-specific urethritis (NSU)

Q What is NSU?

A In NSU or non-specific urethritis, patients complain of pain and discomfort on passing urine and yet microscopic tests and culture for gonorrhoea show negative results. The most common causative germ is *Chlamydia trachomatis*, followed by *Ureaplasma urealyticum*. Infection with one predisposes the patient to infection with the other.

Q How is NSU treated?

A Tetracyclines are usually effective against both the bacteria which commonly causes NSU and are therefore the drugs of choice.

Syphilis

Q What is syphilis?

A Syphilis is a venereal infection caused by a funny-looking corkscrew-shaped bacteria called *Treponema pallidum*. On a lighter note, remember these names. What with the increasingly popular trend of choosing exotic names for their newborn, you really don't want your friends' daughter to suffer the ignominy of being called Treponema or Neisseria!

Q What are the clinical symptoms of syphilis?

A There are four stages of syphilis infection, each with its own signs and symptoms.

1. Primary syphilis. There is usually a single painless lump (the chancre) at the place where the bacteria enters the skin. This appears 10 to 90 days after exposure. This nodule rapidly becomes hard like a button and develops a smooth base with raised, firm edges. The usual places where these chancres are found are the external genital area, neck of the womb (cervix), mouth and anus. Sometimes, the patient may notice many small chancres which occur more commonly over the vulval region. The chancre usually heals after one month.

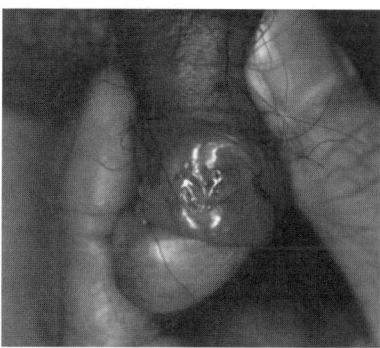

Primary syphilis – chancre of the penis

2. Secondary syphilis. Secondary syphilis usually shows up 3 to 9 weeks after the appearance of the chancre. The features of secondary syphilis are very varied, ranging from widespread rashes typically in the palms and soles, the formation of raised lumps (condyloma lata) in the genital region and other moist areas, and widespread swelling of the lymph nodes.

3. Latent syphilis. This results when the immunity of the body overcomes secondary syphilis. During this stage, the disease is quiet. If left untreated, the patient may suffer from relapses of secondary syphilis or progress to late or tertiary syphilis.

4. Tertiary syphilis. This is the late occurrence of untreated syphilis. The characteristic lesion is a lump called the gumma and the main organs affected are the skin, bones and brain or other internal organs, especially the heart and great blood vessels. The destruction of the heart and great vessels by *Treponema pallidum* becomes manifest roughly 10 to 30 years after the time the bacteria enters the body. The most usual result is a ballooning and weakening of the affected area (aneurysm). When the heart is affected, it becomes less efficient in pumping blood and heart failure soon results. The brain is affected from 2 to 30 years following the primary infection. When this happens, the patient develops headaches, fever, blindness, loss of muscular control when walking and eventually becomes stark raving mad.

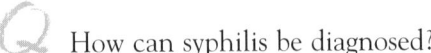 How can syphilis be diagnosed?

Apart from the physical examination, blood tests called the VDRL or TPHA are done. These have only 65 to 85 per cent accuracy as certain conditions like pregnancy, intravenous drug usage and rheumatoid arthritis can give false positive results. The diagnosis can be confirmed by actually taking a scraping from the genital ulcer and examining the organism under a special microscope.

The VDRL and TPHA tests are useful in the follow-up of treatment as falling values of the tests indicate good response to treatment.

Q What is the treatment for syphilis?

A For early syphilis, i.e. primary or secondary syphilis, and latent syphilis of less than a year's duration, benzathine penicillin G is given in the form of a single painful injection. For patients who are allergic to penicillin, erythromycin or tetracycline in tablet form is given. For late syphilis, especially in patients whose brains are affected, the same benzathine penicillin G injection is given weekly for 3 successive weeks. All patients treated for syphilis should have their blood tested 3, 6, 12 and 24 months after treatment. If the results indicate on-going infection or resistant disease, then the patient should be treated with a longer course or with a different antibiotic.

Importantly, the sexual partners exposed to infectious syphilis within the past 3 months should be treated for early syphilis. In patients whose brains are affected, it is necessary to examine the fluid around the brain (cerebrospinal fluid) for bacteria. A sample of the fluid is obtained by carrying out what is called a lumbar puncture. This is done by inserting a needle into a space outside the patient's spinal cord to extract the fluid for examination. Absence of bacteria indicates successful treatment.

Chancroid

Q What is chancroid?

A Chancroid is an STD characterized by the presence of one to three lumps in the genital area appearing 4 to 6 days after exposure. The lumps, sometimes called soft chancres, are small and painful, unlike the chancres in primary syphilis, which are painless. The chancres rapidly break down to become shallow ulcers with irregular edges surrounded by red borders. This bacteria is unable to penetrate intact skin and hence usually attacks areas in which the skin has broken after vigorous sexual activity. This includes areas like the clitoris and lips of the entrance of the vagina (labia). In about 50 per cent of cases, a massively enlarged inflamed lymph node called the bubo develops.

How is chancroid diagnosed?

The diagnosis is usually made by examining the patient and seeing the characteristic chancre or ulcer. This is because the organism which causes the disease, *Haemophilus ducreyi*, is difficult to grow in the laboratory.

How is chancroid treated?

Erythromycin taken orally is the drug of choice, followed by bactrim or amoxicillin. Different strains of *Haemophilus ducreyi* found in different geographical areas show varying responses to antibiotics and if there is no improvement after a week, the drug should be changed. An alternative treatment is the single intramuscular injection of cephalosporin. Healing of bubos is slower than that of ulcers and it may be necessary to have the pus inside aspirated with a sterile needle. Exposed sexual partners should also be treated.

Lymphogranuloma venereum (LGV)

Q What is lymphogranuloma venereum (LGV)? What are the signs of infection?

A LGV is a disease caused by a variant of *Chlamydia trachomatis*. It typically goes through three phases, beginning with the a painless blister, lump or ulcer in the genital area 5 to 23 days after sexual contact. The second phase begins 8 to 30 days later and is characterized by swelling of the lymph nodes, usually on one side of the groin. Fever, headache as well as muscle and joint pains are frequently present. The lymph nodes may then form large abscesses containing pus which eventually drains to the surface.

Q How is LGV diagnosed and how can it be treated?

A An examination of the patient will reveal sores typical of LGV. A blood test called the complement fixation test would confirm the diagnosis. Treatment is with erythromycin tablets taken orally.

Granuloma inguinale (GI)

Q What is granuloma inguinale (GI)?

A GI is an STD caused by a bacteria called *Calymmato bacterium granulomatis*. It is characterized by a painless hard lump followed by the development of a raised red lump in the lips of the entrance of the vagina (labia). These lumps eventually join up and become ulcers. The diagnosis is made clinically by observing the presence of the lumps and ulcers or microscopically by identification of the bacteria (Donovan bodies) in the white blood cells found in the pus.

Molluscum contagiosum

Q What is molluscum contagiosum?

A This is an STD caused by the poxvirus and is characterized by round raised lumps on the skin. These lumps measure 3 to 6 mm in diameter, have a smooth texture like candle wax and may have a central depression. They appear 2 to 8 weeks after infection. The diagnosis is made by seeing the classic lesion.

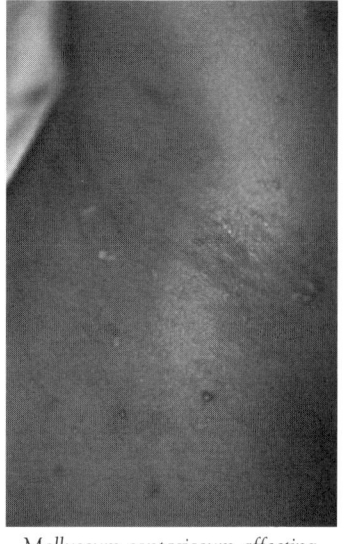

Molluscum contagiosum affecting the armpit

Genital warts

Q What are genital warts?

A Genital or venereal warts (also known as condyloma acuminata) are caused by sexual transmission of the human papillomavirus. They occur mainly on warm, moist areas in the genital region like the entrance of the vagina, the vaginal wall, the neck of the womb and the area around the anus. The spread of the warts is promoted by poor personal hygiene. The warts appear as horny, rough growths which resemble some corals in miniature form.

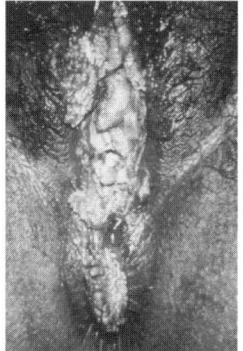 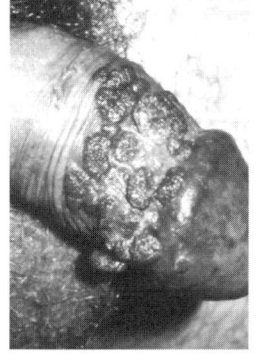 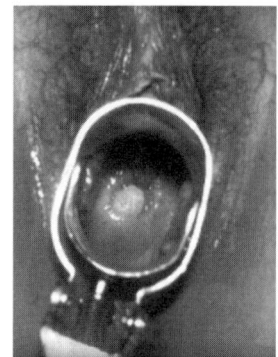

Vulval and anal warts   *Penile warts*   *Cervical warts*

How are genital warts treated?

Genital warts are treated by freezing them using liquid nitrogen (cryotherapy) or using a medicine called podophyllin in a compound tincture of benzoin. The warts are covered with the podophyllin compound with care taken not to touch normal skin. The compound is then washed off in 2 to 4 hours. The podophyllin compound is applied once or twice weekly. If the warts do not disappear after four applications of podophyllin, they should be frozen.

Podophyllin should not be used in pregnancy as it may cause abnormalities of the fetus. Before treating the patient with genital warts, the gynaecologist would need to examine the patient internally using the colposcope to visualize the inner vaginal walls and the neck of the womb. This is important as HPV infection of these areas often leads to precancerous change. Early diagnosis and treatment helps prevent the development of cervical and vaginal cancer.

Precancerous changes

Q What are the delayed effects of human papillomavirus (HPV) infection?

A The HPV attacks cells of the entrance of the vagina (vulva), the inner vagina and the neck of the womb (cervix). The virus enters the cells and affects the DNA of these cells, causing more viruses to be formed, and these in turn affect neighbouring cells. This leads, after many months or years, to abnormalities in the nucleus of the cells which make them prone to cancerous change.

Q How can we tell if the cells are abnormal?

A The abnormal cells can be detected through a Pap smear. In this procedure, the doctor uses a wooden spoon to scrape the surface of the neck of the womb (cervix). This material is then placed on a glass slide and sent to the laboratory. Under the microscope, abnormal cells can be identified and there is a gradation of abnormality from precancer (dysplasia grades 1, 2 and 3) to cancer.

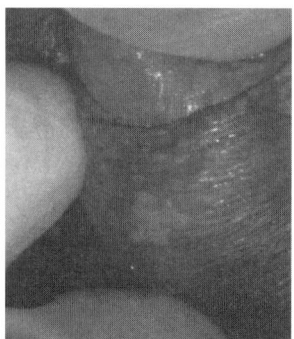

HPV infection of the penis

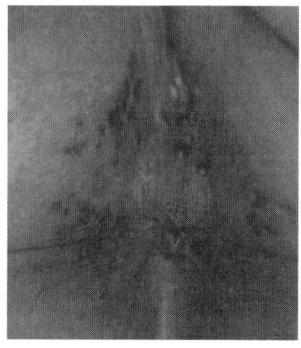

Bowenoid papulosis – an HPV-associated condition

Q Is there a more accurate method for detecting abnormal cells in the vagina or cervix?

A A more accurate and reliable method involves the use of a colposcope. This is a sophisticated optical instrument which allows the surface of the vulva, vagina and cervix to be examined under magnification. The procedure is painless and allows small areas of abnormality, which may be missed in the Pap smear, to be picked up. After applying acetic acid, the abnormal surface appears white with a cobblestone appearance. In more serious cases, abnormal blood vessels are visible. Using a pair of very fine forceps, a tiny piece of tissue is removed and sent to the laboratory for examination. This would enable a precancerous or cancerous condition to be detected early and thus greatly improve the chances of acure.

Q Are there any symptoms in precancerous conditions of the cervix and vagina?

A Precancerous conditions called dysplasia are typically symptomless. The patient feels nothing until an advanced stage is reached, during which there may be bleeding after intercourse or increased vaginal discharge. This underlies the importance of having regular examinations so that early dysplasia can be diagnosed and treated.

Q How are dysplasias of the vagina and cervix treated?

A Being viral in origin, vaginal and cervical dysplasias cannot be treated with the usual antibiotics. The abnormal areas, once identified by the colposcope, have to be physically destroyed using the carbon dioxide laser, or the cryogun (for cryosurgery). Both these procedures are performed on an outpatient basis and are virtually painless.

Given below is a first-person account of a patient who had cryosurgery performed on her:

I had an abnormal class 3 Pap smear. My gynaecologist performed a colposcopy on me and I could see the neck of my womb on a TV screen. It was scary. It appeared red and fearsome, and there were small white patches. He told me he was going to take a small bit of tissue. It felt like a little ant-bite and I bled slightly for 2 days.

A week later, I was back in his clinic and told the good news (I did not have cancer) and the not-so-good news (I had a precancerous condition of my cervix) and I was advised to have cryosurgery. My first question was, 'Do you call it cryosurgery because it is so painful that it will make me cry?' My gynaecologist laughed and said that the procedure was relatively painless and I did not need to stay in hospital.

I agreed and was placed on a couch similar to that used for childbirth. A metal instrument was inserted into my vagina and I heard a hissing noise as he said that the procedure had begun. I felt a dull cramping ache in my lower abdomen as the minutes ticked by. I then felt a warm flush on my face and after what felt like eternity (actually it was only about 5 minutes) he said that it was over and he was going to remove the instrument. I was given two pain-killing tablets and allowed to go home after resting for about half an hour.

The next day, I had a lot of watery discharge from the vagina and had to wear a sanitary towel. This discharge lasted for 10 days. When I returned for the follow-up appointment 2 weeks later, I could see that my cervix was red and inflamed. My gynaecologist explained that this was the normal healing process. Two weeks later, again with the colposcope, I could see that the white patches of abnormal cells were no longer there.

Acquired immune deficency syndrome (AIDS)

Q What is AIDS?

A The acquired immune deficiency syndrome or AIDS is a devastating disease caused by infection with a retrovirus known as the human immunodeficiency virus (HIV). The disease is usually associated with and diagnosed as a result of the appearance of infections and tumours which, otherwise rare, develop as a result of decreased immune function.

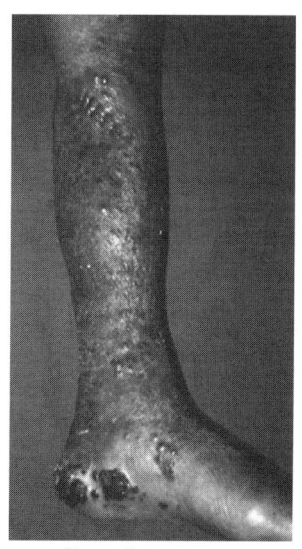

Karposi's sarcoma –
an AIDS-related condition

Q How is AIDS spread?

A Transmission of HIV occurs via the exchange of infected body fluids through sexual intercourse, blood transfusion, the sharing of infected needles by intravenous drug abusers or during pregnancy from infected mother to baby. In the presence of AIDS, other viruses like the *Herpes simplex* virus and the cytomegalovirus become more dangerous and can cause serious widespread infections in the body.

Pubic lice and mites

Q Are there any other diseases which can be sexually transmitted?

A Other less common diseases which can be transmitted sexually are those caused by parasites (colloquially called *kutu*). *Phthirus humanus* (crab lice) and *Sarcoptes scabei* (mites) are insects that may be transmitted through sexual or close contact or through the sharing of contaminated clothes. Sleeping in the same bed with an infected partner makes infestation with these parasites a near certainty.

The bites of these parasites produce an intense and prolonged itch. Pubic lice infestation can be diagnosed by taking a sample of hair from the infected area and examining it under the microscope or colposcope. Nits, faeces (fine red-brown material at the base of the pubic hairs) or the lice themselves (usually also at the base of the hairs) can then be seen. Scabies is most easily diagnosed through the classic burrows which occur in straight lines in the skin, especially between the fingers. By coating the skin with a dark ink, the burrows become more visible.

Q How is crab lice infection treated?

A A thin layer of lindane lotion or cream is applied to the infested hairy area and the surrounding region and then thoroughly washed off after 8 hours. The patient needs to be treated again if lice or eggs are still seen after 7 days. Sexual partners should also be informed and similarly treated. Clothing, towels or bed linen used by the infected person within the past week should be washed with a strong detergent and dried by using the hot cycle of a tumble-drier. Dry cleaning is an effective alternative.

Q How is scabies infection treated?

A Lindane is again used and applied in a thin layer over ALL areas of the body from the neck down and washed off after 8 hours. However, even after effective treatment, the patient may complain of itching for several weeks. If there is no improvement in the clinical condition after a week, the patient would need to be treated again. Further weekly treatments are necessary if live mites are still seen. Sexual partners and close household members are likewise treated. Clothing, especially underwear, towels and bed linen used by the infected person over the last week should be washed with a strong detergent and dried using the hot cycle of a tumble-drier. Lindane should not be given to pregnant women.

Q What about hepatitis B?

A This is another virus which can be sexually transmitted. To date, there is no effective cure for the carrier, who may suffer liver damage and even liver cancer in later life.

Some advice ...

Q Is there any general advice to protect oneself against STDs?

A There are 11 important points to follow:

1. Insist on your partner using a latex condom. As these have smaller pores, they may offer better protection than other condoms.

2. Insist on your partner using a condom EVERY TIME you have sexual intercourse. While there are safe periods for

intercourse if you do not want pregnancy, there are no safe periods for transmission of STDs.

3. Get your partner to put on the condom immediately on erection and not just before ejaculation, after unprotected sexual intercourse has taken place.

4. Roll the condom down all the way to the base of the penis. Some herpes blisters can be hidden by the pubic hair at the base of the penis..

5. Do not use petroleum-based lubricants like Vaseline, which may cause the latex to deteriorate. Do not use saliva for lubrication as it may contain bacteria and spread other infections. The blisters of genital herpes are sometimes found in the mouth. Saliva from an infected mouth can transmit the disease easily.

6. After intercourse, withdraw the erect penis carefully, holding the condom carefully to prevent spillage of semen. This would prevent the spread of STDs, especially gonorrhoea.

7. Get your partner to withdraw promptly after ejaculation so that the condom does not slip off as the erection wanes.

8. Make sure your partner does not reuse condoms.

9. Store condoms in a cool dry place and not for prolonged periods in your handbag. Never use condoms that have been taken out of the glove compartment of a car. Heat can cause the latex to deteriorate.

10. Remember that condoms are only 80 per cent effective in preventing transmission of STDs.

11. I have left the most important golden rule to the last. DO NOT HAVE SEXUAL INTERCOURSE WITH ANY PERSON WHOM YOU SUSPECT MAY HAVE AN STD. The best advice is to be faithful to your spouse and respect the sanctity of marriage.

Losing Control and Regaining It

Child-bearing does wonders to a woman's self-esteem but having to run to the bathroom every time someone tells a joke at a cocktail party is no laughing matter. The inability to control the release of urine is called incontinence and this is closely related to descent (or prolapse) of the womb into the vagina.

Prolapse of the womb and the vagina

Q How many types of womb descent are there?

A There are three types of womb descent. In type 1 (first degree uterine prolapse) the neck of the womb (cervix) is lower down in the vagina than normal. In type 2 (second degree uterine prolapse) the cervix is at the level of the opening of the vagina (the vulva). In type 3 (third degree uterine prolapse) the whole womb, together with the cervix, is entirely outside the vagina.

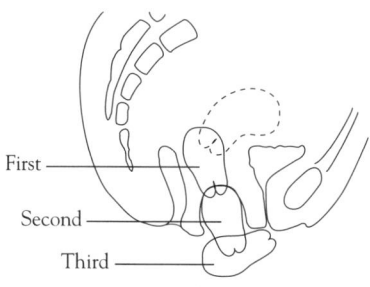

Uterine prolapse – first, second and third degrees

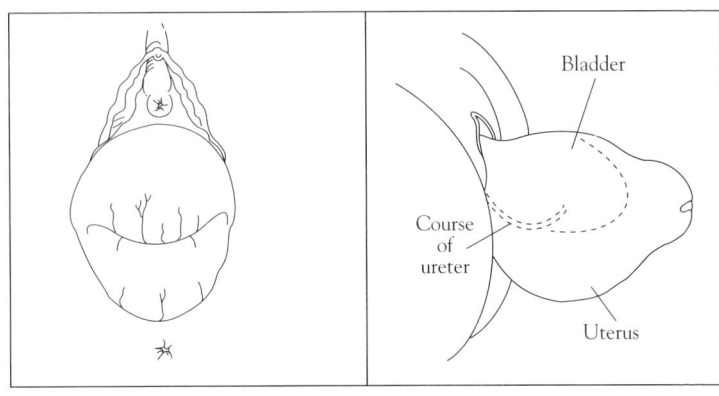

Second degree uterine prolapse –
the cervix appears outside the vulva

Third degree uterine prolapse

Q What causes uterine prolapse?

A Prolapse occurs when the supports of the womb fail. The womb is like the mast of a ship and the guy ropes are the supporting muscles and ligaments. Without the guy ropes, the mast would fall. Similarly, without the support of the ligaments and muscles of the pelvic floor, gravity could cause a woman's uterus to descend as she stands.

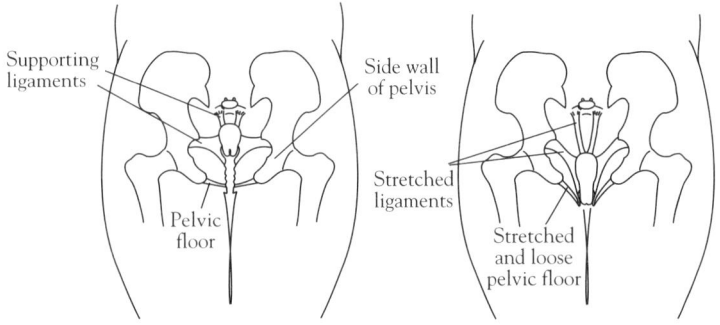

Diagram showing prolapse of the womb

Q   What causes weakness of the supporting structures?

A   The supporting ligaments can be loose following childbirth, owing to an inborn weakness of the tissues or from abnormalities of the spine. However, only a very small proportion of patients suffer from this before pregnancy and childbirth.

Q   How can pregnancy affect the ligaments supporting the womb?

A   The effects of pregnancy on the ligaments are numerous. Firstly, a hormone called relaxin secreted during pregnancy causes a softening of the ligaments and other supporting tissues of the uterus. This allows the ligaments to stretch and therefore accommodate the enlarging uterus as the pregnancy progresses. Secondly, if the labour is long, pressure of the head of the fetus downwards on the muscles and ligaments would cause further stretching of these structures. Permanent damage may then occur.

The third instance occurs in labour when the patient bears down and tries to push the baby out before the neck of the womb is fully open. This means the muscles of the floor of the pelvis are stretched by the full force of the mother's pushing. Also, when the forceps or vacuum is not used properly during deliveries, tears of the vagina or neck of the womb may occur. If these are not properly repaired, permanent damage results. Lastly, during the delivery of the placenta after the birth of the baby, excessive pulling on the cord by an over-zealous doctor may also lead to additional stretching of the supporting ligaments.

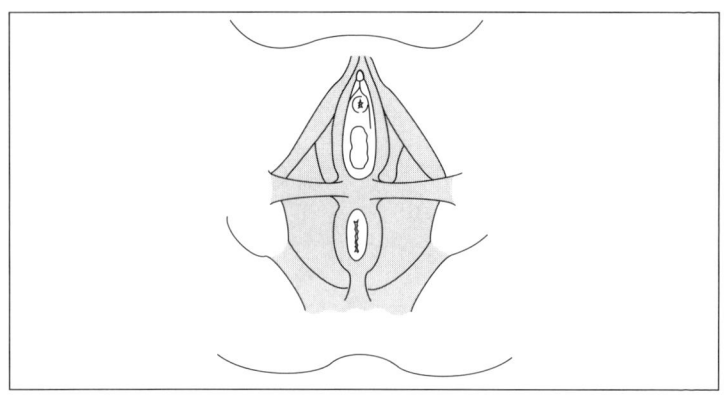

The shaded bands show the muscles of the pelvic floor

Q Are there any other factors which make prolapse worse?

A Apart from the effects of pregnancy and childbirth, other factors can aggravate the situation. Ageing is a significant factor in worsening prolapse. The reduction in the levels of the hormone oestrogen causes a thinning and weakening of the supporting ligaments and muscles of the womb. Other factors are obesity, coughing and chronic constipation. In the latter two situations, there is increased downwards pressure on the womb and this causes further descent.

Q Apart from descent of the womb, is there any other form of prolapse?

A Apart from simple descent of the womb, a loosening of the supporting tissues of the vagina will result in the front wall and/or the back wall of the vagina 'caving' in. A weakening of the upper portion of the back wall of the vagina results in intestines bulging forward (an enterocele) whereas that of the lower part results in the rectum bulging forward (a rectocele). As for the front wall, a protrusion higher up is caused by the bladder bulging inwards (a cystocele) whereas that of the lower portion is caused by the urinary passage or urethra bulging inwards (a urethrocele).

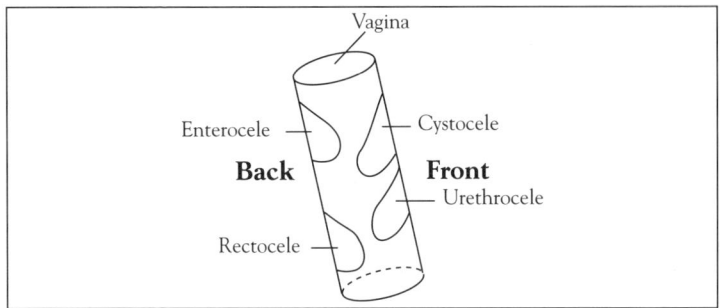

Diagramatic representation of the various forms of prolapse

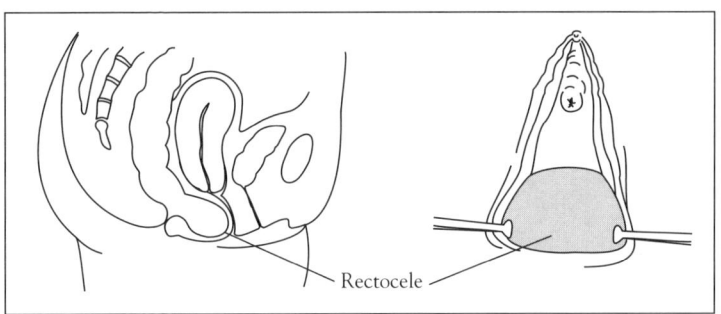

A rectocele

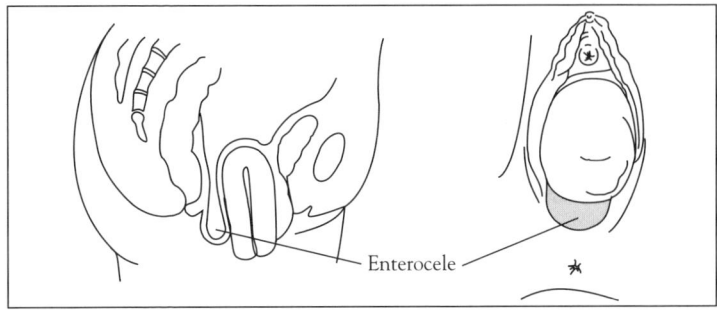

An enterocele

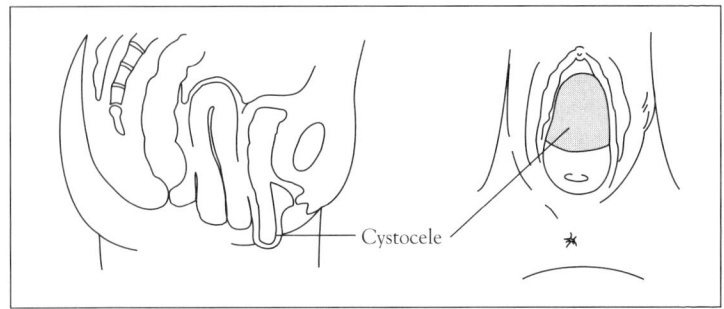

A cystocele

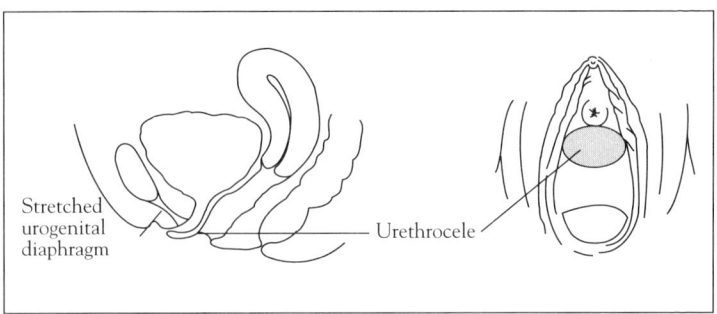

A urethrocele

Q What are the symptoms of womb descent?

A The common complaints are:

1. A feeling of 'something coming down' when the patient is on her feet. This feeling is not there when she lies down.

2. A feeling of always wanting to pass motion. This is caused by the pressure of the lowered womb on the rectum behind it.

3. Backache. This can be caused by a multitude of other conditions but if it is due to the prolapse, the backache will be present only if the patient is on her feet, gets worse as the day goes on and is relieved when she lies down.

4. The feeling of always wanting to pass urine. This is caused by the incomplete emptying of the bladder so that a small pocket of urine remains in the cystocele.

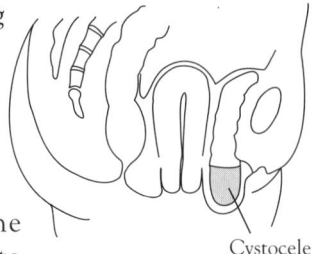

Cystocele

Diagram showing cystocele

5. Pain on passing urine. The stagnant pool of urine tends to become infected, resulting in a burning sensation on passing urine, as well as fever and chills.

6. Uncontrollable leakage of small amounts of urine on coughing, sneezing or laughing.

7. Difficulty in passing urine and passing motion. The former occurs when there is a large cystocele. The patient finds that she is unable to pass urine when the prolapse is down. If she lies down and the prolapse goes back, passing urine becomes possible. The latter is due to the inability to empty the rectum owing to faeces collected in a large rectocele.

8. Sexual problems are common. A very large prolapse would inhibit penetration and extreme laxity of the vagina would make it difficult for both partners to achieve orgasm.

9. Increased vaginal discharge. If there is an ulcer on the protruding cervix, the discharge will be blood-stained.

Treatment for prolapse – non-surgical

Q How can prolapse of the womb and vagina be treated?

A Large prolapses and its effects on the patient can only be corrected by surgery. However, as is commonly the case, the prolapse is minor and this can be corrected through simple measures which do not involve surgery.

What are the methods of treatment which do not involve surgery?

 There are three main methods of non-surgical treatment. These are:
1. Physiotherapy and exercises for the pelvic floor
2. The use of mechanical pessaries
3. Measures to improve the general condition of the patient

 What kind of exercises will help womb descent?

 These are generally exercises to strengthen the muscles of the pelvic floor.

These include pressing together of the buttocks and thighs, holding the tension for 6 seconds and releasing the tension slowly. This is repeated as often as possible when the patient is seated, for example when watching television. This should be done in the comfort and privacy of your own living room and not at a friend's home, lest they think you're a little weird! Stopping the urinary stream mid-way while passing urine is another helpful exercise. Well-motivated patients can also be taught to insert two fingers into the vagina and contract the muscles of the vagina to grip the fingers as tightly as possible. I tell my patients to imagine they have a tail and to try and suck in this imaginary tail and hold it for 6 seconds before relaxing.

The best exercise is one which provides the patient with a direct measure of her progress. An instrument which is used to do this is called Kegel's perineometer. This is a rubber or plastic device shaped like a penis with a basal flange which sits outside the vulva. Inside the perineometer runs a tube which leads to a pressure gauge. The patient can then read off the pressure achieved each time she does her pelvic floor exercises.

Q Is there any other way to exercise the muscles of the pelvic floor?

A For patients who want to be a little different, electrical stimulation of the pelvic floor muscles can be used to improve muscle tone. An electrical current is passed through two electrodes, one placed on the skin of the lower back and another in the vagina. Current is applied in 2-second 'surges', with 2- to 3- second intervals. Treatment is gradually extended to 40 minutes. Any improvement would be apparent after a few sessions and if so the treatment can be continued until the symptoms are relieved.

Q What are pessaries?

A Pessaries are round semi-rigid devices made of plastic, vinyl or polystyrene that come in various sizes.

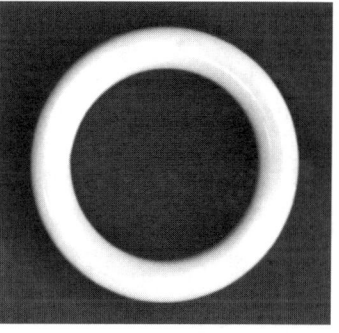

A pessary

They are inserted into the upper part of the vagina around the cervix and work by distending the upper portion of the vagina, thereby supporting the womb and preventing the walls of the vagina from prolapsing.

Q Who should use a pessary?

A The pessary is suitable for a patient who is troubled by the symptoms of her prolapse and is either unwilling or unfit to go for surgery as she may be too old or have numerous other medical problems like heart disease, which would greatly increase the risks of an operation. Sometimes, a pessary can be used as a stop-gap measure to delay operation until a more suitable time, for example, when another pregnancy is anticipated. I once had a 56-year-old lady with a second degree womb prolapse and a large cystocele. She had a ring pessary inserted as she wanted to go on an African safari with a group of close friends before undergoing the operation. She gamely clambered up the Land Rover, which took her over dirt tracks. At the first bump, the pessary fell out and had to be re-inserted by a gynaecologist in Johannesburg.

Q How is a pessary inserted? Is it painful?

A The patient is first asked to empty her bladder (I once had a dear old grandmother spray me with urine from a full bladder as I tried to insert a pessary into her vagina!) and lie on a couch. The pessary is then compressed into a long ovoid shape, lubricated and gently pushed into the vagina where it resumes its circular shape and supports the uterus and vaginal walls. The pessary must not be too tight. The correct size of pessary to use is learnt through experience.

Q What if the pessary is too small or too large?

A A pessary that is too small will soon fall out with the patient sheepishly bringing it back to the clinic in a plastic bag. A pessary that is too large will cause discomfort and difficulty in passing urine or motion.

Q Are there any disadvantages in using pessaries?

A Pessary use increases the amount of vaginal discharge. It also needs to be changed every 4 to 6 months and this may be a bit of a bother. An ill-fitting pessary can cause discomfort, constipation, pain on passing urine and pain on intercourse. If too tight or left in position for too long, ulcers may develop on the vaginal walls and these may become infected. In rare instances, these ulcers may become cancerous.

Q What sort of general measures are useful in treating prolapses?

A The two common conditions which aggravate the problems associated with prolapse, especially stress incontinence, are obesity and a chronic cough. Obesity weakens the muscles for bladder control and if an obese woman can shed 25 per cent of her weight, she can be confident of definite improvement. Similarly, a chronic cough should be treated and if the woman smokes, she should discard her cigarettes immediately. She should also avoid constipation by consuming a high-fibre diet and eating more fruits and vegetables.

Stress incontinence

Q What is stress incontinence?

A As medical students, we all used to troop into the toilets just before the doors of the examination halls opened in March every year. That, we joked, was REAL stress incontinence! On a more serious note, genuine stress incontinence is the uncontrollable leakage of small amounts of urine during episodes of raised abdominal pressure such as coughing, laughing or sneezing.

What causes stress incontinence?

 In general, stress incontinence occurs when there is weakness of the muscles supporting the lower part of the bladder. This can happen following damage sustained during childbirth, when there is prolapse of the bladder or urethra, or the effects of ageing. This results in the lower part of the bladder sagging down and this is seen as the cystocele or urethrocele. During coughing or sneezing, there is a sudden rise in pressure in the abdomen and this serves to propel urine out of the bladder through the urethra. A muscular valve (the sphincter) normally prevents leakage under these circumstances. Sagging or weakening of the bladder and urethral supports results in weakness of this valve. Hence the bladder is unable to hold the urine, which therefore escapes.

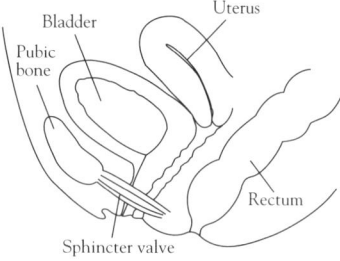

Diagram showing the sphincter mechanism for control of urination

 How can stress incontinence be treated?

 Mild cases of stress incontinence can be treated by general measures such as weight reduction and the treatment of chronic cough and constipation. Pelvic floor exercises (Kegel's exercises) are also useful in strengthening the sphincter muscles at the base of the bladder. Should these simple measures fail, then a surgical procedure called a Kelly's stitch is done.

Q What is a Kelly's stitch?

A A Kelly's stitch is a relatively painless operation which is done under general anaesthesia. The patient is placed flat on her back with her legs drawn up. The genital area is then cleaned with an antiseptic solution and the operating field covered with a sterile cloth. Urine is drained from the bladder using a metal tube and the bulge in the front vaginal wall (the cystocele) is then visualized. A cut is made in the vagina directly over the cystocele until the cystocele is freed and can be pushed upwards.

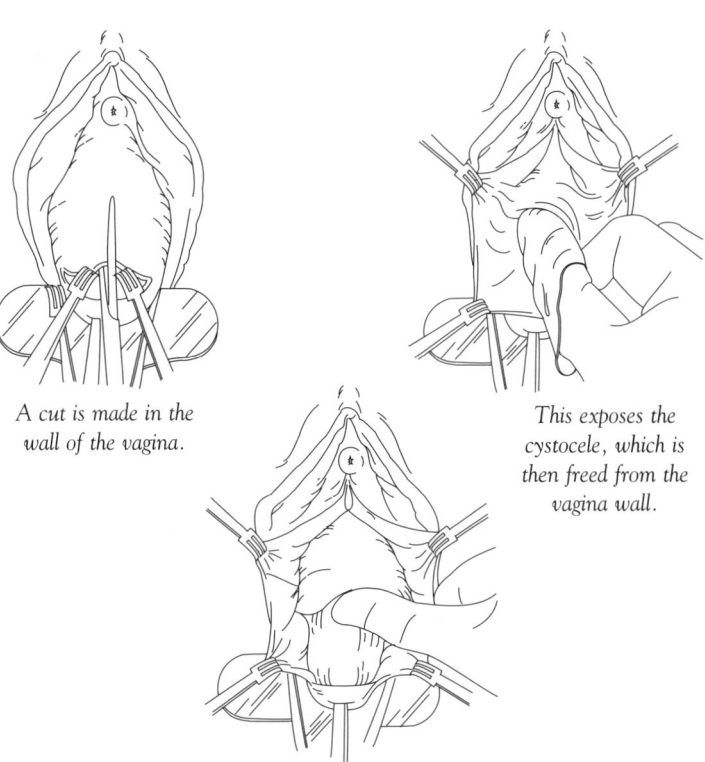

A cut is made in the wall of the vagina.

This exposes the cystocele, which is then freed from the vagina wall.

The cystocele is pushed upwards.

The base of the bladder is then supported by three strong sutures (the Kelly's stitch), which are fastened at the side to the undersurface of the pubic bone.

In this way, the valve at the bladder neck is strengthened and the urinary passage (the urethra) lenghtened. Both have the effect of preventing involuntary leakage of urine when the patient exerts violently as in coughing and sneezing. The excess loose skin of the vaginal wall is then cut off and the edges sewn together.

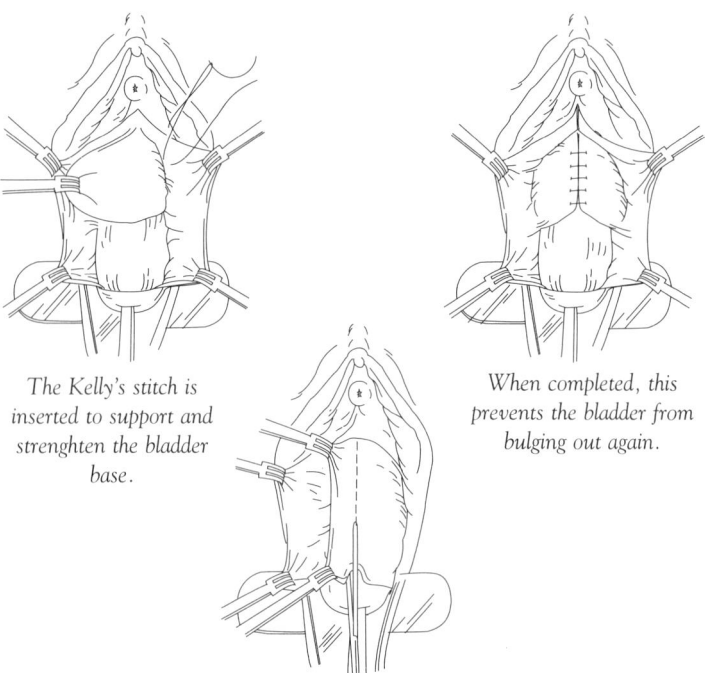

The Kelly's stitch is inserted to support and strenghten the bladder base.

When completed, this prevents the bladder from bulging out again.

Excess loose vaginal tissue is cut away and the cut edges are stitched together.

At the end of the operation, the vagina is tightened in front and the bulge in the front wall of the vagina no longer exists. Given below is a first-person account:

It all started 20 years ago after the birth of my fourth child. Brian was a big baby then (Just as he is now!) weighing in at 10 pounds. It was a labour I want to forget as I had died a thousand deaths waiting for him to be born.

A month after the delivery, I had trouble holding my urine. It got steadily worse until last week when I wet the back seat of my friend's car as she went over one of those wretched speed-reducing humps on the road. My gynaecologist explained the reasons why my bladder was weak and also what the whole operation was going to achieve. It made a lot of sense and I agreed.

My enthusiasm disappeared when I was placed on that cold operating table with the bright lights above me. I almost chickened out when they stuck some discs on my chest to check my heart. Before I knew it, the anaesthetist had given me an injection on my hand. I felt a blackness come over me and the next thing I knew, I was back in the ward.

My bottom felt sore and very full. My gynaecologist explained that there was a long piece of gauze inside to prevent any bleeding. I also felt like passing urine all the while but was told that it was unnecessary and the feeling was caused by a rubber urine tube placed inside my urinary passage. I was quite uncomfortable the whole night but luckily there was not much pain.

The next morning, the nurse woke me up at 6 a.m. to sponge me. Soon, my gynaecologist came and to my great relief, removed the cloth in my vagina. That took away much of my discomfort. That evening, the rubber urine tube was taken off and I was advised to pass urine every hour before the bladder became too full. I got a fright initially as I found it very difficult to pass urine as compared to the past years and had to sit down and strain for 10 to 15 minutes. My gynaecologist explained that it was because the bladder muscle was not used to the tighter outlet and I had to let it build up its strength. Also, he explained that there was some swelling from the operation which made it more difficult to pass urine and that this swelling would soon subside. He was right as I was able to pass urine quite easily after a week and best of all, I did not 'leak' anymore.

My husband and I have just signed up for ballroom dancing classes, something which I have always wanted to do but did not dare to. Soon you'll see me tripping gracefully across the dance floor, with little fear of dripping like before!

Q   Are there any complications from this operation?

A   Apart from the possibility of the usual anaesthetic complications, there may be excessive bleeding or infection after the operation. There is a small possibility of inability to pass urine if the bladder neck is over-supported or if the bladder muscles are too weak. However, this condition can be treated by leaving the rubber tube in for a longer period, sometimes up to a week, to allow the swelling from the operation to subside. The difficulty in passing urine eventually passes without further treatment.

Q   What can be done if this operation still fails to cure incontinence?

A   Another operation called the Aldridge sling can be done. This is a more painful operation as it involves cutting through the skin of the lower abdomen. Using the patient's own tissue, a sling is fashioned and is used to support the base of the bladder and the urethra.

Q   What are the possible complications from this procedure?

A   As this is a more complex operation, the potential for complications are somewhat higher. Apart from the complications of the Kelly's sling, there may be more bleeding as well as infection of the wound in the abdomen. The base of the bladder and the urethra may be damaged at the time of surgery. Also, retention of urine, if it occurs, tends to be more serious and troublesome.

Q Besides stress incontinence, are there any other types of urinary incontinence?

A Apart from stress incontinence, there are three other types of urinary incontinence: urge incontinence, overflow incontinence and true incontinence.

Urge incontinence

Q What is urge incontinence?

A In urge incontinence, the patient develops a powerful desire to pass urine and needs to run quickly to the nearest toilet. This usually occurs with a full bladder and may be triggered off by a sudden movement. Unlike stress incontinence, larger amounts of urine are passed. There may also be pain on passing urine.

Q What causes urge incontinence?

A This is caused by 'instability' of the bladder muscles rather than a mechanical cause as in stress incontinence. The instability of the bladder muscles causes them to be 'irritable', contracting at the slightest stimulation. Sometimes, there is also infection of the bladder, which contributes to its irritability. When there is infection, there is pain on passing urine.

Q How can we diagnose urge incontinence?

A The first step in diagnosis is to carry out tests to exclude any medical condition which affects bladder control. This includes diseases which affect the nervous system, like Parkinson's disease and diabetes. The urine is also examined to exclude urinary infection as a cause of the irritable bladder. Thereafter, a test called cystometry is performed. This is done in the clinic as an out-patient procedure. Using an instrument called a cystoscope, the surgeon examines the inside of the bladder for stones or tumours. A bladder filling and voiding test is then carried out. The bladder is filled with saline and the pressure recorded at intervals. In urge incontinence, the pressure inside the bladder is higher than normal and the bladder muscles tend to contract when it is filled to a lower volume than normal bladders.

Q How can we treat urge incontinence?

A The first step in the treatment of urge incontinence is to carry out complete tests to exclude any underlying condition which needs to be separately treated. The urine is sent for examination and culture and any infection of the bladder treated with the correct antibiotics. In some instances, urge incontinence is the manifestation of tuberculosis of the kidneys.

Having confirmed urge incontinence, the patient is taught the 'bladder drill'. In this procedure, the patient is kept in hospital and taught to pass urine by the clock, regardless of whether she feels like doing so or not. Starting at half-hourly intervals, the time between emptying is increased half-hourly daily until intervals of 3 or 4 hours. This 'teaches' the nervous system and the bladder muscles how to hold the urine and prevents voiding at inopportune times.

Q Are there any drugs which help urge incontinence?

A A mild sedative is used in conjunction with the bladder drill and this increases its success. A drug called oxybutinin is also given 3 times a day and this works by decreasing the sensitivity of the bladder muscles.

Overflow incontinence

Q What is overflow incontinence?

A Overflow incontinence occurs when the bladder is filled so much with urine that it becomes over-distended. The distension then causes the neck of the bladder to open up, allowing passage of urine into the urethra.

Q What causes overflow incontinence?

A Overflow incontinence is caused mainly by diseases which affect the nervous system, so that the patient does not feel like voiding or is incapable of doing so. Examples of diseases which cause nerve damage are diabetes and Parkinson's disease. Others, like senile dementia or tertiary syphilis, makes the patient incapable of voiding. Sometimes after delivery, injury to the urethra causes urinary retention and the bladder is then distended to the point of overflow.

Q How is overflow incontinence treated?

A The underlying cause has to be identified and treated. For urinary retention after delivery, a rubber catheter is inserted into the bladder, allowing the urine to drain over a few days. This enables the bladder muscles to regain its tone and on removal of the catheter, normal voiding function would have been re-established.

True incontinence

Q What is true incontinence?

A This is the constant leakage of urine due to an abnormal connection (a fistula) between the cavity of the bladder and the exterior.

Q What causes true incontinence?

A Damage to the bladder wall or urethra during a difficult operation to remove the womb or during childbirth is the commonest cause of true incontinence. Radiation damage to tissues following radiotherapy for conditions like cancer of the cervix is a possible cause but is rare now, owing to the very precise dose calculations in radiotherapy for cancer.

Q How do we treat true incontinence?

A Small fistulas connecting the bladder to the vagina would close spontaneously upon draining the urine continuously with a catheter. This can be inserted either through the urethra or through the skin of the lower abdominal wall using a suprapubic catheter. Larger fistulas or those that do not close spontaneously with a catheter need to be surgically repaired.

12   On Golden Pond

This is the most exciting time of a woman's life. The children have grown up (presumably well!) and are happily married. The office is running smoothly, with competent junior staff at the helm, and the bank book shows a healthy balance. It is the time to lie at the helm, back, relax and take holidays. The management of problems after cessation of the menstruation (menopause) is therefore of paramount importance in enabling the woman to enjoy a healthy, active life-style.

Menopause

Q   What is the menopause?

A   The menopause is the time when a woman stops menstruating, owing to hormonal changes following ageing of her ovaries. It can only be said have happened after 12 months without menstruation.

Q   What is the usual age of menopause?

A   The average age of menopause is 51 years. It varies from population to population, from 42 years in poor countries to 53 years in more affluent communities. This is because good nutrition and good health prolongs the reproductive life-span of a woman. Other factors which influence the age of menopause are body weight, exercise and smoking. The latter decreases the age of menopause.

What is perimenopause?

This is the period of time around the menopause, in which marked changes in the menstrual cycle occur. These changes are usually accompanied by a variety of symptoms which characterize the menopause.

Problems with the menopause which require treatment

Problems of ...	Result in ...
The blood vessels	Hot flushes and night sweats
The urinary and genital systems	Thinning of the vaginal wall Vaginal infection Difficulty in controlling urine Repeated bladder infections Irregular or heavy bleeding
The mental state	Vague complaints of a lack of well-being Depression Anxiety, panic attacks Joint and muscle pains

Problems with the menopause which need to be prevented

Problems of ...	Result in ...
The heart	Chest pains (angina pectoris) and heart attacks
The bones	Thinning of the bones (osteoporosis)
The brain	Strokes, Alzheimer's disease

Hot flushes

Q What do hot flushes feel like?

A Patients complain of a burst of heat lasting 2 to 5 minutes, often accompanied by profuse sweating. The skin feels warm and the skin on the head, neck and chest reddens. The heart beats noticeably faster and palpitations are also commonly felt. Sometimes the patient wakes up with a strange feeling at night, just before the hot flushes occur.

Q How common are these hot flushes?

A These symptoms, usually mild, are present in 30 to 50 per cent of women aged above 40 years with regular menstrual cycles. At the time of menopause, 80 per cent of women experience hot flushes and 35 per cent consider them distressing. Thereafter, the frequency of hot flushes decline slowly and by the age of 60, only 35 to 40 per cent of the women still experience them.

Q When do these hot flushes start and how long do they last?

A In most women, they start years before and lasts for years after the natural menopause. They begin at a younger age in women who smoke and are still commonly present after 60 years. The most severe hot flushes usually occur within a certain period – ranging from 3 months to 3 years – after the last menstrual bleeding.

Q   What causes hot flushes?

A   The exact mechanism is not definitely known. It is believed that a decrease in the influence of hormones produced by the ovaries causes improper activation of the heat loss mechanism of the skin. This leads to dilatation of the blood vessels and increased sweating.

Q   How can this be treated?

A   Hot flushes can be treated with oestrogens, other hormones like progesterone, special breathing techniques, exercise and a drug named clonidine.

Q   How effective are hormones in the treatment of hot flushes?

A   Oestrogens are effective in treating hot flushes and night sweats especially if these are frequent and severe. These are given in the form of the combined oral contraceptive pill. Progesterone compounds have also been found to be effective but these need to be given in large enough daily doses.

Q   Are there any side-effects of hormone treatment?

A   Side-effects may be experienced and these include nausea, headaches, irregular vaginal bleeding, a tingling sensation of the nipples and a feeling of general bloatedness.

Q   How long should the hormones be taken?

A   Hormonal treatment of hot flushes and night sweats should continue for at least 2 years. If complaints return after treatment is stopped, then the medication should be continued for another year.

Q   What drugs can be used?

A   A drug called clonidine is useful in treating hot flushes. This is taken twice a day. Side-effects include sleepiness and dryness of the mouth and nose.

Q   What if a patient is unable to take hormones?

A   Paced breathing techniques are useful in controlling hot flushes. The patient is taught how to breathe slowly and relax the various muscle groups in the body and this has been found to be effective in reducing hot flushes in 50 per cent of women suffering from them.

Changes in the urinary and genital organs

Q   What are the effects of the menopause on the urinary and genital organs?

A   The lowered oestrogen levels after the menopause causes thinning of the lining of the entrance of the vagina (vulva), the inner vagina and bladder, and a decrease in the blood flow to these organs.

Q   What does the patient feel in this instance?

A   She experiences vaginal dryness and irritation, or alternatively an increase in vaginal discharge and itchiness, pain or bleeding after intercourse and 'looseness' of the vagina. Problems with passing urine are also common.

These include increased frequency of urination and pain on passing urine, waking up at night to pass urine, an uncontrollable urge to pass urine and frequent repeated attacks of bladder infection.

Q How common are urinary problems after the menopause?

A Although not many patients complain of this, 10 to 15 per cent of postmenopausal women experience severe inability to control their urine daily. Repeated bladder infections are also a major problem in elderly women.

Q How do we treat vaginal problems?

A The hormone oestrogen forms the mainstay of treatment. This is preferably given through the vagina so that the hormone can act directly on the tissues. This takes the form of vaginal tablets or an oestrogen-containing vaginal ring that is left in place for 3 months. Oestrogen in the form of a vaginal cream is also available and this is applied twice a day to the vulva. This would cure most of the burning and itching sensation caused by thinning of the vaginal walls due to the lack of oestrogens.

Q Are there any other ways in which oestrogens can be given?

A A skin patch containing oestrogens can be applied to the skin, through which the hormones are absorbed into the blood circulation. Oestrogen tablets can also be swallowed daily but these may cause nausea and headaches in sensitive patients.

Q How long should treatment be carried out?

A For dryness and thinning of the vagina, improvements may show after several weeks although the maximum benefit is not seen until months later. Painful intercourse usually improves only after 6 to 12 months of treatment.

Q Does oestrogen treatment reduce the chance of getting infections of the bladder and vagina ?

A Oestrogen treatment reduces the incidence of infections of the bladder and vagina by promoting the growth of 'friendly' bacteria, making it more difficult for disease-causing germs to grow. It also causes the walls of these organs to become thicker and more healthy. For the prevention of recurrent infection, treatment should be carried on for life.

Bleeding in the perimenopausal period

Q What is the significance of bleeding problems in patients close to the menopause?

A Bleeding problems become more common in women above the age of 40 years. In general, frequent but regular bleeding or regular cycles with decreased bleeding indicate a hormonal imbalance. These are less serious than irregular bleeding, which usually results from a more sinister cause, like cancer of the womb. The causes of bleeding problems during the perimenopausal period can be summarized as follows:

1. **Hormonal imbalances**
   Too little oestrogens

2. **Diseases of the genital organs**
   Non-cancerous growths of the neck of the womb (cervical polyps)
   Infections of the neck of the womb (cervicitis)
   Non-cancerous growths of the womb (endometrial polyps)
   Abnormal thickening of the lining of the womb (endometrial hyperplasia)
   Fibroids of the womb
   Enlargement of the womb (adenomyosis)

3. **Cancerous conditions**
   Cancer of the neck of the womb (cervical cancer)
   Cancer of the body of the womb (endometrial cancer)

4. **Problems with pregnancy**
   Impending miscarriage
   Ectopic pregnancy

5. **Problems with the blood clotting system**
   Lack of clotting factors
   Leukaemia
   Low blood platelet count

6. **Other illnesses**
   Thyroid disease
   Liver disease
   Kidney failure

7. **Bleeding due to medication**
   Drugs to dissolve blood clots in the body (anticoagulants)
   Prolonged steroid treatment
   Chemotherapy for cancer treatment
   Drugs for epilepsy
   Dialysis

Q What is the most common cause for irregular bleeding from the vagina?

A Hormonal imbalances and benign growths of the neck of the womb (cervical polyps) are the commonest non-cancerous causes for irregular vaginal bleeding. Infections of the neck of the womb (cervicitis) or polyps in the womb are also quite often encountered in clinical practice.

Q What about fibroids?

A Fibroids are present in the womb in a third of all perimenopausal women. Although these fibroids may be silent and not cause any problems, those that lie just next to the lining of the womb are usually the cause of abnormal vaginal bleeding.

Q What is the most common age for developing cancer of the womb?

A Precancerous changes of the womb (endometrial hyperplasia) is seen mainly at 40 to 50 years and overt cases of cancer of the womb at 50 to 70 years.

Q Can a woman get pregnant during the perimenopause?

A This is uncommon but can happen. In fact, the *Guinness Book of Records* puts the oldest mother at 56 years! Fertility declines rapidly after 40 years but if a pregnancy occurs, it is likely to lead to complications. At the age of 45 years, a woman has a 50 per cent chance of suffering a miscarriage.

Q What other diseases can cause abnormal bleeding?

A 50 per cent of women with thyroid disease can have abnormal bleeding, usually in the form of heavy menstruation. Liver and kidney diseases can also lead to a change in bleeding patterns. Women who are on progesterone-only hormonal contraception can also experience irregular bleeding owing to fluctuating hormone levels.

Q How can abnormal bleeding be treated?

A Firstly, the abnormal heavy bleeding must be stopped. This can be done by giving the patient progesterone tablets. The bleeding usually gets less within 9 to 16 hours and stops within 2 days. Treatment should be for at least 10 days to stabilize the lining of the womb. If this fails, then a dilatation and curettage (D & C) of the womb under anaesthesia may be necessary.

Q Is there any chance of a recurrence?

A If any of the above conditions such as thyroid disease or fibroids of the uterus exists, they must first be treated to prevent a recurrence of the abnormal bleeding. Having excluded a separate treatable disease, the patient may require hormonal treatment for a couple of years in order to prevent recurrence of dysfunctional bleeding. Hormone treatment is also useful in preventing hot flushes, bone loss, dryness of the vagina and heart disease.

Q   What sort of hormones can be used? Are there any side-effects?

A   Combined oral contraceptive pills are the drugs of first choice in the treatment of perimenopausal bleeding. The oestrogen component has the additional benefit of preventing problems due to low oestrogen levels such as vaginal dryness and frequency in passing urine. Side-effects are an increase in weight, abdominal discomfort, irregular vaginal bleeding and tenderness of the nipples. Most of these complaints disappear after the first 4 months of treatment.

Progesterone in tablet form can also be used from days 16 to 25 or from days 5 to 25 of the menstrual cycle. Treatment should be continued for at least four cycles to allow the lining of the womb to stabilize but there is a 25 per cent recurrence rate after the treatment ends. By taking progesterone tablets daily, most women will stop menstruating but the main disadvantage of this treatment regimen is the occurrence of small irregular amounts of vaginal bleeding and periods of unpredictable blood flow.

Q   What if a patient cannot take hormones?

A   Drugs known as prostaglandin-synthetase inhibitors, which are commonly used for muscular pains, can be given for women intolerant to steroids. These cause a marked reduction in menstrual blood loss and need be taken only during menstruation. In addition, they lessen menstrual pain (dysmenorrhoea). Unfortunately, these drugs do not work for patients with fibroids of the womb and cause gastric pains, headaches, nausea and vomiting in sensitive patients.

Are there any other alternatives?

 Antifibrinolytic drugs like tranexamic acid causes a reduction in heavy menstrual blood loss by 40 per cent and are useful for patients who cannot take oestrogens.

Another drug called danazol can reduce menstrual blood flow by 70 per cent but the side-effects are bloating, weight gain, rash on the body, nausea and muscle cramps. When on danazol treatment, a patient needs to be on a form of contraception like the condom to prevent pregnancy as this drug can cause abnormalities in the baby.

A third form of medication is the GnRH analogue which has been described previously in the treatment for endometriosis. They are very effective in controlling heavy bleeding but can bring about hot flushes, pain during sexual intercourse and a generalized feeling of irritability. Thinning of the bone may also occur if treatment is carried out for more than 3 months. Treatment using GnRH analogues is also very costly.

What if medication cannot control the bleeding?

A range of operations are then necessary to stop the bleeding. This includes dilatation and curettage (D & C) of the womb to remove the thick lining of the womb responsible for the heavy bleeding. Benign growths of the womb (polyps) can also be removed during the D & C. The tissue removed in the procedure is then sent to the laboratory for examination to rule out cancer as a cause for the abnormal bleeding. Although blood loss may be reduced in the first cycle postoperatively, it will usually return to preoperative levels after 4 months.

Another operation aims to destroy the lining of the womb, which is the source of the bleeding. This procedure is called endometrial ablation and is carried out using a hysteroscope. This is a metal tube which is inserted into the neck of the womb and through this tube the inner surface of the womb can be seen. The lining of the womb can be cut and removed (resected), burnt or destroyed using laser. This procedure is painless as it is done under general anaesthesia. In about 80 per cent of cases this successfully stops the bleeding.

If all else fails, surgery to remove the womb (hysterectomy) would be necessary to stop the heavy bleeding. This procedure is relatively safe, with a mortality rate of 7 in 10 000 cases. However, some pain after the operation is inevitable. Also, women who have their womb removed because of abnormal vaginal bleeding may experience other menopausal symptoms like hot flushes at an earlier age.

Other common complaints

Q What other complaints are common around the menopause?

A Many women also experience mood changes around the menopause. These include vague complaints of a lack of well-being, depression, anxiety, irritability, joint and muscle pains and thinning of the skin, especially around the mouth and eyes. These women usually have a decreased interest in social events, family and friends and their behaviour becomes generally less friendly. Emotions, feelings, libido and sensations head South and generally women feel more nervous, tense and depressed. A recent survey of post-menopausal women revealed that they suffered from the following symptoms:

Other common complaints

Tiredness	50%
Muscle/joint pain	45%
Headache	30%
Sweating	27%
Sleeplessness	25%

 What aggravates these complaints?

 Usually, well-adjusted women regard hot flushes and the other common problems of the menopause as part and parcel of life and tolerate them well. It is only when these symptoms appear too early or last way beyond the menopause that they feel out of control, depressed and anxious.

How can these symptoms be treated?

Hormone replacement therapy (HRT) with oestrogens often leads to an improvement in mood within 3 months of initiating treatment. As for joint pains, symptoms usually disappear in a quarter of the women within 3 months of starting hormone therapy and the symptoms improve in a further 45 per cent.

Oestrogen therapy is also useful in the treatment of dry mouth, a burning feeling of the tongue, and an altered sense of taste, which sometimes occurs in the postmenopausal woman.

Heart disease

Q What is the risk of suffering from heart disease after the menopause?

A Diseases of the heart and blood vessels (cardiovascular diseases) is the leading cause of death in women in Singapore, America and Europe. After the menopause, the risk of cardiovascular diseases increases dramatically.

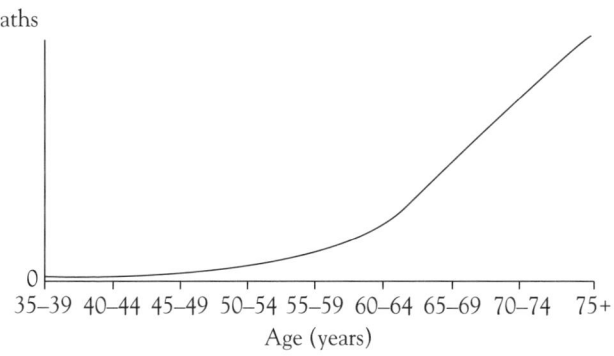

Deaths from cardiovascular diseases by age group

Q How does menopause cause an increase in heart disease?

A Heart and vascular disease is caused mainly by deposits of cholesterol and related substances (atheroma or atheromatous plaques) on the walls of blood vessels, making the vessels narrower. This narrowing impedes the distribution of blood and when heart vessels are significantly blocked, chest pains on exertion (angina pectoris) are felt. In more severe blockages, a heart attack (myocardial infarction) will follow.

After the menopause, the blood cholesterol level is raised together with that of low-density lipoprotein. This accelerates atheroma formation. At the same time, the levels of high-density lipoprotein, which protects or delays atheroma formation, is lowered. An amino acid in the blood called homocysteine has also been shown to cause the early development of heart disease and abnormalities in the blood vessels of the brain and heart. Blood levels of homocysteine are raised following the menopause.

Lastly, the ability of the heart to contract to pump blood is less efficient after the menopause. This, coupled with the increased resistance to blood flow in the narrowed blood vessels and an increase in the ability of the blood to clot after the menopause, predisposes the elderly woman to heart disease.

Hormone replacement therapy (HRT)

Q What is the role of hormone replacement therapy in the prevention of heart disease after the menopause?

A Taking oestrogens after the menopause reduces the relative risk of heart disease. Studies have found a 35 per cent reduction in the incidence of heart disease in women who have been on or are currently on oestrogen replacement therapy as compared to postmenopausal women who have never been on such treatment. The beneficial effect is more pronounced in women who are currently on hormones as compared to those who took hormones in the past. The death rate from heart disease in patients who were on HRT was also reduced.

Q What about progesterone therapy?

A Progesterone has often been prescribed together with oestrogens in postmenopausal HRT to reduce the risk of cancer of the womb due to the unopposed effect of oestrogens on the lining of the womb. Unfortunately, progesterone reduces the beneficial effect of oestrogens in protecting against heart disease as it tends to raise the level of low-density lipoprotein (the bad guy) and lower the level of high-density lipoprotein (the good guy) in the blood.

Q Who should take oestrogens after the menopause?

A Women with existing coronary heart disease or those with an early onset of the menopause as a result of surgery or cancer treatment with drugs (except breast cancer) would definitely benefit from oestrogen therapy. Postmenopausal women who are at a higher than normal risk of developing heart disease because of a raised blood cholesterol or low-density lipoprotein level should also take oestrogens. Lastly, women who have diabetes, high blood pressure and a family history of heart disease or raised blood cholesterol level would also benefit from such treatment.

Q How are the oestrogens taken and for how long?

A The oestrogens need to be taken in tablet form once every morning for 5 or more years for their beneficial effect to be sustained. Although oestrogens have a definite beneficial effect on the heart, their side-effects must also be considered. However, it is widely accepted that the advantages of oestrogen therapy far outweigh the disadvantages, especially when one considers the improvement in the quality of life oestrogens bring. It is, however, important to keep in mind that assessments based on the 'average' woman may not apply to an individual with a different risk-benefit profile. The decision to take oestrogens or otherwise after the menopause is a very personal one and this should be decided by the patient in close consultation with her doctor, taking into account the patient's own personal risk factors and outlook in life.

Q Does oestrogen therapy help in a woman's mental function?

A Oestrogen treatment is widely believed to have some beneficial effect on a woman's memory and logical thinking after the menopause. This in itself leads to better self-esteem and a happier outlook in life. Here is a first-person account of a 51-year-old woman who underwent hormone replacement therapy:

It started a year ago as a weird feeling. I could not put my finger on it. I did not feel like doing anything. I was no longer interested in my usual activities like mahjong and the usual hen parties. Even the birth of my first grandchild did not seem too exciting. My husband and children encouraged me to take up some hobby but I just was not interested.

Lately, sex also became a torture. I was very dry and my vagina felt like sandpaper whenever we had intercourse. I did not dare tell my husband because of the many stories I have heard of men having mistresses. Also, I was going to the toilet more often. The last straw was when I woke up in the middle of one night feeling that my pyjamas were full of ants. I quickly changed and checked my pyjamas. There was nothing on them and yet I still felt like there were ants crawling on my skin.

I went to see my gynaecologist, who took my blood pressure, examined my breasts and did a Pap smear. He then suggested some hormone tablets. At first I was reluctant as I was afraid of side-effects but he reassured me that it was generally safe and that we could just try it out for 3 months to see if I felt better. I agreed and started taking these red tablets, one a day for 3 weeks. After 2 weeks, I began to feel much better. I was more energetic and I did not have to go to the toilet as often. Also, I did not find sex as painful. I have started going out more often. After one month, not only do I feel better but my friends also say I look better!

 Are there women who should not take oestrogens after the menopause?

 There are four groups of women who should not take oestrogens. These are:

1. Women who have had breast cancer
2. Women who have had cancer of the womb
3. Women with severe liver disease
4. Women with a rare blood condition called porphyria

Oestrogens promote the growth of breast cancer cells and in women who have had the tumour before, HRT may cause a recurrence of the disease. Similarly, the cancer cells of the womb are oestrogen-dependant and hence the hormone should not be used in these patients. The liver is the organ that breaks down oestrogens, hence in severe liver disease, oestrogens should not be used as they would tax the failing liver.

 What about progesterone?

 Patients with brain tumours called meningiomas should not be given progesterone as the hormone may result in a rapid enlargement of the tumour. The use of progesterone may be considered if the condition has been stable for many years without signs of recent growth of the tumour. Even then, the progesterone should be given only for a few days in a month and even then at very low doses.

Osteoporosis

Q What is osteoporosis?

A Osteoporosis is thinning of the bones and results in a lower bone density. Bone loss with ageing is a universal phenomenon resulting in a lower bone mass and disordered bone architecture. This in turn increases the risk of fractures. The bone loss which ultimately results in osteoporosis begins when the menstrual cycle starts to become irregular during the years approaching the menopause. Interestingly, women who experience frequent night sweats tend to lose more bone mass.

Q How common are fractures in the elderly woman?

A After the age of 50 years, a woman has a 30 per cent risk of suffering from a fracture of the bone of the spine (vertebrae), an 18 per cent risk of sustaining a hip fracture and a 14 per cent risk of a wrist fracture in her lifetime. These risks are increased if the woman is thin, smokes, does not exercise and has a family history of such fractures. Women who have had a stroke before, those with poor eyesight or those on medication for high blood pressure have a tendency to fall and these women are particularly at risk.

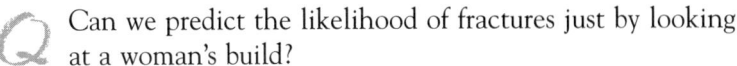

Q Can we predict the likelihood of fractures just by looking at a woman's build?

A To some extent, the likelihood of a woman developing osteoporosis and subsequent fractures can be assessed by her external appearance. There are three main groups:

1. The woman who is thin above the waist but has heavy buttocks (pear-shaped body)

2. The woman who is uniformly fat (an orange-shaped body)

3. The woman who is uniformly thin (Olive Oyle-shaped body, named after Popeye's girl friend)

All factors being equal, the pear-shaped body has a lower risk of fractures as the fat in the buttocks is a good storage medium for oestrogens which help increase bone mass. The woman who is uniformly fat is also protected against osteoporosis but the general obesity poses other health hazards like an increased risk of heart disease. The woman who looks like Olive Oyle may not be a likely candidate for heart disease but her overall thinness results in a decreased storage capacity for oestrogens and hence puts her at an increased risk of developing osteoporosis and fractures.

Q How can osteoporosis be diagnosed?

A Osteoporosis can be diagnosed by performing X-rays on the spine. This method can detect the condition only after there is 30 per cent bone loss. A more accurate and sensitive method is a procedure called X-ray absorptiometry. During this procedure, the patient lies on a table and a beam is passed over the body. An instrument called a photon counter is used to measure the bone mass. This is a very safe procedure which does not require injections, sedation or fasting.

Q   Can hormone replacement therapy prevent osteoporosis?

A   When taken for 5 years or more soon after the menopause, oestrogen therapy reduces the risk of subsequent osteoporosis-related fractures by 50 per cent. When women who have had their ovaries surgically removed because of disease were treated with oestrogen for more than 10 years, the bone mass of the spine was found to be 32 per cent higher and that of the long leg bone (femur) 12 per cent higher than that in untreated women. In women with natural menopause, oestrogen treatment has the same beneficial effect on bone mass. Unlike in the case of heart disease, progesterone treatment does not nullify the effect of oestrogens on the skeleton. On the contrary, progesterone compounds actually enhance the effect of oestrogens on the skeleton, thereby causing a significant increase in general bone mass.

Q   Is there any other way to prevent osteoporosis?

A   Prevention of osteoporosis can largely be achieved by adopting an active life-style. Medical evidence has shown that definite protection against osteoporosis and fractures is achieved if a woman is on her feet for at least 4 hours a day as the effect of gravity and weight-bearing enhances bone mass. Even non-weight-bearing exercises like swimming and water ballet are beneficial. Stopping smoking also helps tremendously in preventing osteoporosis.

Q   How about in cases of established osteoporosis?

A   Oestrogen therapy has a definite beneficial effect in women with proven osteoporosis. Studies have shown that oestrogens given through the skin with added progesterone increases the average vertebral bone mass by more than 6 per cent and decreases the fracture rate by 45 per cent.

Q How are the hormones given?

A Oestrogens in adequate doses can be taken orally or are given through a skin patch, gel, cream or injected just under the skin. In addition, progesterone is added in tablet form and this enhances the effect of oestrogens in increasing bone mass.

Q Are there any other drugs which help prevent osteoporosis?

A Besides oestrogens, calcium and vitamin D in the form of tablets also help increase bone mass. The hormone calcitonin is given either by injection or as a nasal snuff to prevent osteoporosis. Anabolic steroids, besides destroying the careers of many world-class athletes, are also effective in building up bone mass.

Q When should treatment begin and how long should it last?

A HRT should begin at the menopause and continue indefinitely for maximum protection against fractures. This is especially so in cases where bone spectrophotometry shows a very low bone mass. Even if treatment is not life-long, a 5-year duration of oestrogen therapy will reduce the fracture rate by half.

Strokes

Q What are strokes?

A A stroke is a term used to describe the condition in which blockage of a major blood vessel in the brain leads to a severe impairment of a person's muscular and mental functions. If the blockage is severe, death can occur. The blockage of the blood vessel, like that of the vessels of the heart which leads to heart attacks, is commonly caused by atheromatous plaques of cholesterol compounds which harden and narrow the arteries.

Q How common are strokes after the menopause?

A Stroke is one of the leading causes of death for post-menopausal women in Singapore, America and Europe. A 50-year-old woman has a 22 per cent chance of developing a stroke in her lifetime and a 10 per cent chance of dying from it.

Q What are the effects of HRT on the development of strokes?

A Blood flow to various parts of the brain is increased by oestrogen therapy after the menopause. This also results in a one-third reduction in the risk of developing a stroke and a two-thirds reduction in the risk of dying from a stroke. The addition of a progesterone compound does not modify the beneficial effects of oestrogens.

Alzheimer's disease

Q What is Alzheimer's disease?

A This is a form of mental derangement. Such a person gradually loses all his mental faculties such as memory, reasoning, recognizing people and surroundings until ultimately a vegetative state is reached and they are unable to take care of themselves. Dementia due to Alzheimer's disease is a common disorder with a profound impact on the quality of life not only of the individual but also for the family members. There is a genetic element in the development of Alzheimer's disease. That is to say, if one parent had Alzheimer's disease, then the chance of the children developing it is higher.

Q What is the effect of hormones on Alzheimer's disease?

A There is substantial medical evidence to suggest that oestrogen use may prevent or at least delay the onset of Alzheimer's disease in the postmenopausal woman.

Cancer

Q Does HRT increase the risk of a woman developing cancer?

A The risk of developing cancer of the womb is increased in women if they have had oestrogen-only HRT for more than 10 years. That for cancer of the breast is increased after more than 5 years of oestrogen-only HRT.

Q   How can deaths from these cancers be reduced?

A   Early detection is the key. For cancer of the womb, frequent sampling of the lining of the womb as an out-patient procedure (endometrial sampling) is useful in detecting precancerous changes. Once detected, treatment with oestrogens is stopped and progesterone is given to reverse the abnormal changes in the lining of the womb. For breast cancer, monthly examination of the breasts is useful so that lumps can be detected early. Mammograms and ultrasound examinations are also done periodically to pick up early cancerous changes.

13 Finer Points about the Birds and the Bees

In my practice, I notice a steady decline in the age at which girls become sexually active. These are changing times and there is a pressing need for proper sex education in the schools as well as the home. At dinner the other night, a friend of mine related this hilarious story. She is the mother of two boys aged 12 and 10. The elder son had just had a talk on sex education in school and had come back thoroughly disgusted. He approached his parents and said, 'We just learnt how babies are made. It's so gross! I can't believe you and Dad actually did that. The thought of it makes me want to throw up. And to think you did it not just once but twice!'

Sexual response in men and women

Q What is sexual stimulation?

A Sexual stimulation involves the activities which lead to a sexual response in the man and the woman. This can be brought on by touch, hearing, taste, smell and sight. For example, a woman may derive erotic stimulation from seeing her partner in the nude, hearing his voice, listening to a particular type of music, or smelling bodily odours or a favourite cologne. Some men are sexually stimulated by tasting saliva or genital secretions.

Q How important is touch in sexual stimulation?

A Touch is arguably the most important stimulus in evoking the normal sexual response. Certain areas of the body are called 'erogenous zones' as they are exceptionally sensitive to touch and the promotion of sexual arousal.

Q Where are the erogenous zones in a man?

A Erogenous zones in the man include the lips, the neck and the area around the genitalia, especially the tip of the penis (glans penis), the scrotum and the inner thighs.

Q Where are the erogenous zones in the woman?

A These include the lips, breasts (especially the nipples), neck, genital region (especially the clitoris) and the inner thighs. Other areas include the inner aspect of the elbows, knees and wrist.

Q What are the stages of the male sexual response?

A There are three phases of the male sexual response: penile erection, ejaculation of semen and then resolution.

1. The erection phase. This is the initial phase of the male sexual response and is characterized by erection of the penis due to an increase in blood flow to the organ. This phase is rapid and in younger men can occur in the space of a few seconds. Occurring simultaneously are other reactions. A slight discharge escapes from the tip of the penis. The skin of the scrotum contracts, becomes thick and loses its baggy, wrinkled appearance. The testes also

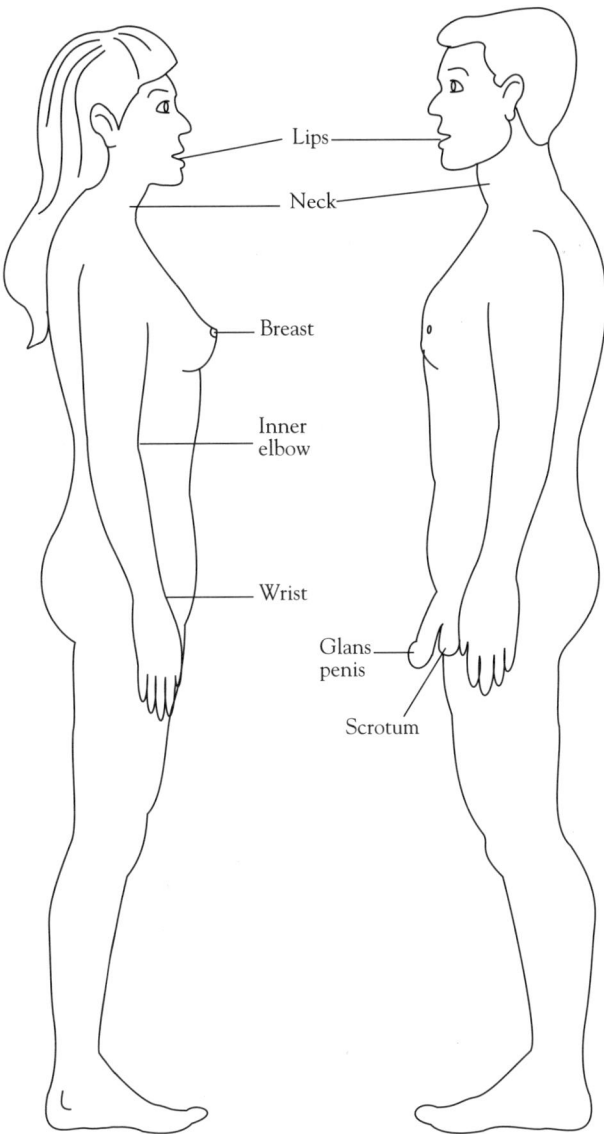

Lips

Neck

Breast

Inner
elbow

Wrist

Glans
penis

Scrotum

Erogenous zones in a woman and a man

rise within the scrotum and increase in size by between 50 and 100 per cent. The muscles of the body become more tense and the blood pressure, heart rate and breathing all increase. The nipples become erect and the skin takes on a flush.

2. The ejaculation phase. The bodily changes of the erection phase increase in intensity until the ejaculation phase is reached. This comprises two components, namely the emission phase and the expulsion phase. In the emission phase, contractions of the internal sex organs like the seminal vesicles, prostate gland, testes and vas deferens cause semen to be carried to the entrance of the urethra.

    During the expulsion phase, rhythmic contractions of the muscles of the penis force the semen to spurt out of the penis at regular intervals of about 0.8 seconds. At this moment, the man experiences the intense pleasure of orgasm.

    A refractory period then follows, during which the male cannot respond to further sexual stimulation. For a variable length of time, he is unable to become erect or ejaculate again. The duration of this refractory period increases as the man grows older.

3. The resolution phase. During this phase, the sexual organs gradually return to their unstimulated state. For the penis, this occurs in two stages. Just immediately after ejaculation half the erection is lost quite rapidly. The rest of the erection then dissipates more slowly over about 20 minutes. The scrotum becomes wrinkled and baggy again and the testes return to their original unstimulated size and position. The changes in blood pressure, heart rate and breathing subside and perspiration occurs.

What is the female response cycle?

 There are also three phrases in the female sexual response:

1. The phase of increased vaginal wetness and swelling. This initial phase in the female sexual response is caused by the swelling and engorgement of blood vessels of the genital region similar to the phenomenon of penile erection in the male. The inner two-thirds of the vagina enlarges and the outer third becomes so engorged and swollen that the opening of the vagina becomes much narrowed. This is what Masters and Johnson, two well-known sex researchers, call the 'orgasmic platform'. Next, there is an increase in clear, odourless vaginal discharge and this occurs within 20 to 40 seconds of sexual stimulation.

   At the same time, a change in the colour in the labia occurs as a result of the swelling of blood vessels. In women who have never given birth before, the opening of the vagina turns from pink to bright red. The colour changes are less vivid in women who have had babies previously. In these women, the labia changes from red to a deep burgundy. This colour change always occurs before the woman experiences orgasm and once this colour change has occurred, then orgasm would follow if there is sustained sexual stimulation. During an advanced stage of sexual arousal, the clitoris becomes engorged and swollen and retracts behind a fold of skin above the clitoris (the clitoral hood).

   The uterus also swells because of an increase in blood flow. Increases in muscle tension, pulse rate, breathing and blood pressure occur as in the male. However, in the female sexual response, nipple erection and flushing of the skin is much more marked. This is called the 'sex flush' by

Masters and Johnson and it appears like a rash which begins under the ribs and quickly spreads upwards to the breasts and other parts of the body.

2. The orgasm phase. The changes which take place during the initial phase of sexual stimulation increases in intensity until the phase of orgasm is reached. During this time, there is marked contraction of the muscles of the genital organs similar to that which takes place during the expulsion stage of ejaculation of the male sexual response. Stimulation of the clitoris is the main factor which triggers off the orgasm phase.

Strong spasms of the orgasmic platform, the pelvic muscles and the uterus occur in a series of 3 to 15 rhythmic contractions which commence at intervals of about 0.8 seconds and thereafter diminish in intensity and frequency. These contractions are accompanied by a generalized increase in muscle tension throughout the body and an intense feeling of pleasure.

Unlike in the man, there is no refractory period following orgasm in the woman and she is able to experience a series of orgasms separated by intervals of only a few seconds between them. If sexual stimulation is maintained, this can continue until the woman becomes exhausted.

3. The resolution phase. During this phase, should sexual stimulation continue, repeated orgasms are possible. However, at this stage, the man would probably have ejaculated and the refractory period of the male sexual response would have begun. Likewise, the female body returns to its normal unstimulated state. The orgasmic platform rapidly loses its swelling and the changes in the

colour of the labia quickly vanishes. The rest of the vagina and the uterus take a further 15 to 20 minutes to return to its original size.

Thus, like in the man, the resolution phase of the woman takes place in two stages. The first phase which involves the muscles of the genital organs (the orgasmic platform) occur quickly. The second phase is the gradual shrinkage of the rest of the vagina and the uterus, and this takes place more slowly. Associated with the second slower phase is the gradual return of the blood pressure and heart rate to normal levels, with the appearance of a thin film of perspiration over much of the body.

Sexual dysfunction in women

What are the common forms of female sexual dysfunction?

These can be summarized as follows:

Problems with arousal or the initiation of intercourse
Inadequate sexual interest
Abnormality of the lubrication–swelling phase
Spasms of the vaginal muscle (vaginismus)

Problems with orgasm

Problems with sexual pleasure
Inadequate sexual pleasure
Painful intercourse (dyspareunia)

Inadequate sexual interest

Q Is the lack of sexual interest abnormal?

A The level of sexual interest considered normal varies from couple to couple. Most couples experience periods when they become disinterested in sex. This happens during times of illness, fatigue or mental stress. I once had a new bride complain to me saying that her husband, after their honeymoon, had totally lost all interest in her. At a separate consultation, I found out that the husband, a salesman, had been told by his superior that he would lose his job if his sales did not double in the next 3 months. Such temporary losses in sexual interest are not considered to be abnormal and usually no treatment is necessary. Moreover, there are many happily married couples who do not consider sex to be an essential element in their relationship. In such a situation, both husband or wife do not find prolonged periods of sexual abstinence to be a problem.

On the other hand, a lack of sexual interest in one partner may be poorly accepted by the other. There then exists a strong reason for marital discord and treatment for the condition becomes necessary. A lack of sexual interest may exist alone or with some other sexual problem. Some women who have no interest in sex and who will not initiate it themselves will nonetheless enjoy intercourse when it has been initiated by their spouses. They are capable of getting sexually stimulated when the erogenous zones are touched and are also capable of experiencing multiple orgasms.

What is the 'normal level' of sexual activity?

 In my practice, this varies from having intercourse twice a day in young couples to once a month for those more advanced in years. On the average, most couples have intercourse 3 times a week.

What are the causes of a lack of interest in sex?

A number of possible causes exist. Hostility, resentment or anger towards her spouse is perhaps one of the commoner causes for a woman's lack of interest in sex. In such a situation, the loss of interest is restricted only to sex with the spouse.

Another common cause is the psychological barrier to sexual intercourse which arises from a previous bad experience. For example, a woman who had a harrowing sexual experience as a young girl would find the thought of sexual intercourse threatening and she would anticipate pain before the act actually begins.

A repressive upbringing where sex is a dirty word and not freely discussed may also inhibit the normal sexual response in the woman.

Yet another cause would be general debilitating illnesses such as kidney disease, diabetes or medication for high blood pressure. Past operations like removal of the womb (hysterectomy) or breast (mastectomy) might contribute to a low sexual interest.

The next cause is depression, which usually occurs in perimenopausal women. At this time, the children have grown up and the husband may be too engrossed in his job or on the golf course (the 'empty nest syndrome').

Lastly, inadequate sexual interest may be the result of deficient or inadequate stimulation. I find this a common problem among my patients. After a few years of marriage, the husband takes the wife for granted as a 'sex object'. Gone are the roses, chocolates, soft music and gentle caresses. Gone also are the days when he tells her how beautiful she is. Instead the whole sex act is over before she actually gets into the lubrication phase. No wonder the woman begins to lose interest in sex!

 How can a woman's interest in sex be improved?

Open communication between husband and wife is crucial. Any marital discord must be dealt with squarely and open dialogue usually solves a problem before it blows out of proportion. The woman must tell her husband what her problem is so that he would be aware and become sensitive to her needs. Any previous bad experience must be vocalized and brought into the open so that it can be dealt with. Systemic illnesses should be treated. Sometimes, a woman loses her sexual drive when she is on the oral contraceptive pill. As such, another form of contraception should be used.

Lastly, I usually tell the husband in private that a little tenderness would oil the wheels of their marriage. Treat her like he did when they were courting. The little notes, the compliments and the tender pecks on the cheek act as an important prelude to actual love-making. More foreplay with caresses of the erogenous zones would increase his partner's sexual pleasure and greatly increase her desire for sex.

Abnormality of the lubrication-swelling phase

Q What kind of abnormality can occur with the lubrication-swelling phase?

A In cases of dysfunction of the lubrication-swelling phase, the increase in vaginal secretions, the swelling of the inner two-thirds of the vagina and the formation of the orgasmic platform do not occur normally. This can be compared to failure to get erect in the male but the consequences are fortunately much less disastrous. Many women with this kind of dysfunction lack erotic feelings and do not undergo the lubrication–swelling phase of the normal female sexual response but a number of these women are still able to reach orgasm during sexual intercourse.

Q Is this a serious problem?

A Yes and no. This problem may be experienced in all sexual activities or only in some of them. For example, a woman may have lubrication problems only with her husband, towards whom she harbours negative feelings. The effects of these women's impaired arousal on men are also varied. Some do not mind their wives behaving like cold fish. Others find it deeply distressing and see the lack of sexual gratification in their wives as an adverse reflection of their own sexual prowess. Not uncommonly, this lubrication-swelling failure occurs when the humdrum routine of marriage settles in after the initial sexuality.

Q What are the causes of lubrication-swelling failure?

A Diseases which cause lubrication-swelling failure are those that lead to decreased vaginal secretions. A major cause is the decrease in oestrogen levels following the menopause. Diabetes, which affects the nerves necessary for the increase in vaginal secretions during sexual stimulation can lead to vaginal dryness. Mental factors like stress are also important causes.

Feelings of rejection, anger or hostility would easily lead to lubrication–swelling failure in the woman. I once had a husband complain to me that he found intercourse with his wife painful as the entrance to her vagina was always dry even during intercourse which took place every Sunday night. The reason became apparent when I found out that he spent Mondays to Saturdays with his mistress.

Vaginismus

Q What is vaginismus?

A Vaginismus is the strong contraction of the muscles of the outer third of the vagina which occurs involuntarily when the woman perceives the threat of vaginal penetration. When this happens, insertion of the penis into the vagina is naturally prevented. Sexual intercourse becomes impossible without great difficulty and pain. In more severe cases, the thigh muscles are involved, so that the legs are clamped together in a vice-like grip, and the back arched backwards.

Apart from these muscular contractions, a strong psychological component exists in the woman with vaginismus. She has an almost pathological fear of vaginal penetration. Sexual gratification can be attained by fondling the clitoris and normal orgasm is possible provided there is no threat of vaginal penetration. Severe cases of vaginismus commonly reaches the courts as non-consummation after many years of marriage.

Q Is vaginismus a common problem?

A Vaginismus constitutes approximately 10 per cent of cases of female sexual dysfunction.

Q Is this a serious problem?

A Yes, in that the sufferer experiences a whole range of negative feelings from that of anxiety and humiliation to inadequacy and disappointment as she finds herself unable to enjoy normal sexual relations with her husband. If the problems persists for any length of time, the woman would soon develop fears of her partner deserting her for someone more co-operative. Another common anxiety is the failure to conceive and these additional mental stresses usually only serve to compound the problem.

The husband of a woman suffering from vaginismus usually tends to be more timid and subservient than normal and as such is usually likely to perpetuate the problem. He then feels frustrated and disappointed and often imagines that he is a failure as a lover. If this denial of sexual intercourse becomes prolonged, then immense psychological stresses would arise in the male and he may develop sexual dysfunction himself.

What are the causes of vaginismus?

Most commonly, the woman would have experienced a painful and unpleasant sexual experience earlier in her life. Although these unpleasant conditions no longer exist, she is still mentally very fearful and continues to respond to the threat of vaginal penetration with a reflex protective response.

Another cause of vaginismus is an excessively repressive upbringing. Sometimes, a family background in which sexuality is considered to be dirty, sinful and contrary to orthodox religious beliefs causes the patient to grow up with the fear of even washing her own genitals. This has been shown to play a significant role in the development of vaginismus.

At other times, it is the fear of contracting a venereal disease or an unwanted pregnancy that triggers off vaginismus. This problem becomes ingrained if the fear is not quickly rationalized and dealt with.

A large proportion of women suffering from this condition are also misinformed about sexual matters and it is this ignorance that leads to their fear of vaginal penetration. For example, some sex researchers have found that many women with vaginismus believe that the hymen is like a Rock of Gibraltar that completely obstructs the vagina and that breaking it would lead to a great deal of pain. Hence their reaction to attempts at vaginal penetration.

Lastly, vaginismus is found in some women with a lesbian tendency. They are dysfunctional towards sexual relationships with men but are perfectly comfortable and relaxed when being intimate with other women.

Q How is vaginismus treated?

A Vaginismus can be treated by dilating the vagina under anaesthesia. In this way, the muscle spasm associated with the condition is overcome. The second method employed with some success is hypnosis, during which the patient is made to realize that sexual intercourse need not be painful but is instead pleasurable.

Problems with orgasm

Q What is orgasm failure?

A In this kind of sexual dysfunction, the woman is unable to produce the involuntary reflex muscular contractions of the genital muscles which are necessary for attaining orgasm. This is similar to the inability to ejaculate in the man. This condition may occur on its own or may co-exist with another form of sexual dysfunction. For example, some women have a great interest in sex and are able to achieve a high level of sexual excitement but are just unable to reach the point of orgasm. Many such women are actually quite happy with their sexual status as the high level of sexual excitement achieved is able to provide them with a great deal of pleasure even though orgasm always escapes them. On the other hand, some women with orgasm dysfunction may feel frustrated and this would often then affect her partner, who would to some extent blame himself for her failure to climax.

Q How often does orgasm failure occur?

A It is common for a newly married woman not to experience an orgasm during the initial months of her sexual initiation. Studies have shown that the proportion of women who have never experienced an orgasm during sexual stimulation decreased from 26 per cent in the first year of marriage to 10 per cent by the twentieth year. For individual couples over a short span of time, it is common for the woman not to attain orgasm every time there is sexual intercourse. This is especially so if the man rushes through the whole act before the woman can get sexually stimulated.

Q What causes failure to have an orgasm?

A The nature of the sexual stimulation plays an important role in the attainment of orgasm by the woman. Some women are unable to climax with penile thrusting alone but are able to do so if there is manual stimulation of the clitoris. Needless to say, insufficient sexual stimulation would lead to failure to have orgasm. The mental state of the couple is also important. Relaxed, sensitive love-making rarely fails to be completely satisfying for both the man and the woman whereas failure to experience an orgasm is common if the pressures of the office are brought into the bedroom.

Another reason for orgasm dysfunction is pain on intercourse. This can occur when the vagina is dry from inadequate lubrication or if there is vaginal or vulval infection. An interesting association with orgasmic dysfunction is a poor father-daughter relationship in a very sexually repressive upbringing. This may lead to the woman putting a lid on her sexual feelings and thus inhibiting orgasm for fear of ridicule when it occurs. Lastly, failure to have an orgasm may be an outward manifestation of a systemic malady like diabetes or kidney disease.

Q Is a failure to reach orgasm a serious problem?

A This depends very much on the couple. I have seen many couples as patients who enjoy a very satisfying sex life and have babies without the wife ever experiencing orgasms. On the other hand, I have also seen strapping, macho men extremely distressed over their wives' inability to climax as they find it a slight on their masculinity. When this happens, it is not uncommon for the wives to be similarly disturbed. They would complain that there is 'something missing' in their sex lives and if the problem persists, they may begin to lose interest in sex.

Q How can this condition be treated?

A Firstly, any underlying disease must be treated. The couple must then be taught how to relax and it must be impressed on the woman that it is common not to attain orgasm every time they make love. This would be largely effective in removing any mental stress which would compound the situation. Lastly, the most effective means of sexual stimulation for the woman is employed, be it fondling or oral stimulation of the clitoris. Once there is adequate sexual stimulation for an effective length of time, orgasm usually follows. Once it has been attained, the re-enactment of successful intercourse should not be too difficult.

Painful intercourse

Q What is dyspareunia?

A Dyspareunia is also known as painful sexual intercourse for the woman and this can occur at the time of initial penile penetration, during or after the event. The pain may originate from the entrance of the vagina (the vulva), the pelvic muscles or the vagina itself. Dyspareunia may exist in isolation or in conjunction with other forms of sexual dysfunction. If the woman has pain on intercourse for any period of time, she would soon lose interest in sex and develop problems in lubrication and orgasm.

Q   What causes dyspareunia?

A   The commonest causes of painful intercourse can be traced to the entrance of the vagina. These include problems with the hymen which may be too rigid or imperforate from birth or scarred following childbirth. Infection of the Bartholin's gland located at the lower portion of the vagina or vaginismus itself can give rise to dyspareunia. Sometimes, the entrance to the vagina (the vulva) can become irritated and inflamed from over-zealous cleansing or from sensitivity to detergents or certain fabrics in the underwear.

Pain in the vagina is usually the result of insufficient lubrication either from a lack of oestrogens after the menopause or from vaginal infections.

Occasionally, the patient complains of a deep internal pain on penile thrusting. This can arise from a womb that is tilted backwards (retroverted uterus), an ovarian cyst, endometriosis of the pelvis or a fibroid of the uterus.

Q   Can mental conditions cause dyspareunia?

A   Apart from the physical conditions described above, mental stress may cause dyspareunia. Hostility or anger towards the man may lead to insufficient lubrication and hence painful intercourse.

Q How can we treat dyspareunia?

A The first step is to identify the cause of the painful intercourse. Simple surgery helps in cases of rigid or imperforate hymens. Vaginal infections can be treated with the appropriate antibiotic or antifungal agent. Cysts of the Bartholin's glands can be surgically drained or removed. In the event of poor lubrication following the menopause, oestrogen treatment would alleviate the condition. For deep internal pain, especially that arising from a womb that is tilted backwards, adjusting coital position would be useful. Pelvic endometriosis, ovarian cysts or large uterine fibroids can be surgically removed. Mental factors of hostility or anger need to be resolved before sexual intercourse becomes pleasurable again.

Sexual dysfunction in men

Q What are the causes of diminished sexual interest in the man?

A A man may lose interest in sex because of a number of causes. It may be the result of an underlying illness like diabetes or cardiac disease or, more commonly, mental factors. Problems in the office or unpaid bills at home often dampen the desire for sexual relations. Once again, the low level of sexual interest may or may not pose a problem in the marriage.

A few years ago, a couple consulted me as they had waited 3 years for a baby. On enquiring about their sexual habits, I realized that they had never had intercourse and were totally ignorant of the birds and the bees! They thought that babies were made by literally just sleeping together (and waiting).

The closest they ever got to love-making was a gentle good night peck on the cheek. This lack of sexual interest in both the man and the woman was well-accepted in each partner and there was no marital discord.

Q What is the commonest male sexual dysfunction?

A In my practice, impotence or erectile problems is the commonest form of male sexual dysfunction.

Q What is impotence?

A Impotence is the impairment of erectile function. This means the inability of the man to achieve and maintain an erection long enough for intercourse to take place.

Q What are the common causes of impotence?

A Common causes of impotence include systemic illnesses like kidney or liver diseases, previous operations especially around the genital area such as operations on the prostrate gland, and various drugs.

Q What sort of drugs can cause impotence?

A These include sedatives, medication for high blood pressure and drugs used in the treatment of mental illnesses.

Q Can mental factors cause impotence?

A The erectile phase of the male sexual response is extremely sensitive to mental stresses. Anxiety during love-making is a common cause of impotence. The fear of impotence feeds on itself and the problem usually worsens if the couple still attempt to make love when there is erectile failure.

Q   What is premature ejaculation?

A   Premature ejaculation is the lack of sufficient voluntary control over ejaculation of semen during sexual intercourse.

Q   What causes premature ejaculation?

A   Unlike impotence, where there usually is an organic cause, the roots of premature ejaculation are usually psychological. Anxiety and stress reactions are believed to be major causes of premature ejaculation. For example, a man who had a previous experience of premature ejaculation from nervousness may become embarrassed from his wife's ridicule. During the next attempt at love-making, he becomes anxious that a similar occurrence would take place. This imposes considerable stress on him, causing a loss of control and another bout of premature ejaculation.

Q   How is premature ejaculation treated?

A   The treatment basically involves stimulation of the man until an erection is attained but without allowing intercourse to take place. When he feels that ejaculation is about to take place, his wife gently squeezes and draws down lightly on both testicles. This has the effect of preventing ejaculation and is sustained until the feeling of impending ejaculation wears off. The whole process is repeated and the patient is thereby taught control of the ejaculation phase of the male response. This is repeated and actual intercourse is permitted only after he has regained sufficient confidence in controlling the timing of ejaculation.

14

Through the Scope and Under the Knife

Apart from the visit to confirm a much awaited pregnancy, a woman does not usually bounce into my clinic bursting with enthusiasm. The initial conversation often goes like this.

'Good morning, Mrs Tay. And how are you today?' 'When I have to come and see you then it cannot be anything good!' is the usual sardonic reply.

Although the usual gynaecology clinic is not as much a fun-filled place as Disneyland, neither should it be a terrifying House of Horrors. A simple understanding of the nature of the various procedures is usually all that is necessary to make your visit to the gynaecologist a time to look forward to.

The 'scopies'

Recent advances in light physics and the use of fibre optic technology has made it possible for us to use endoscopes to look inside the body. We shall refer to these procedures as the various 'scopies':

The 'scopies'

Colposcopy
Hysteroscopy
Falloposcopy
Cystoscopy
Laparoscopy

Q What is colposcopy?

A Colposcopy is an important procedure used in the diagnosis of precancerous or early cancerous change or infections of the cervix, vagina and vulva. Using a magnifying optical instrument called the colposcope, the cervix is checked for any abnormal change. It is a totally painless procedure and is done with the patient fully awake and without anaesthesia.

When performing a colpo-scopy, the gynaecologist stains the surface of the cervix or vagina with a thin solution of vinegar. This has the effect of causing abnormal cells to turn white. Under magnification, abnormal blood vessels also become visible. Abnormal areas are thus identified. A tiny bit of tissue the size of a grain of sand is taken and sent to the laboratory for examination. The diagnosis of the disease is then confirmed by the pathologist who examines the bit of tissue and determines the nature and extent of the disease.

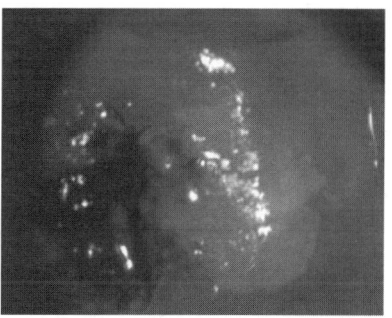

Colposcopy of the cervix. The white patches suggest HPV infection.

Q What is hysteroscopy?

A In hysteroscopy the inner surface of the womb is examined under magnification using an instrument called the hysteroscope. This is a metal tube-like device with a light source at one end and a eyepiece at the other through which the inside of the womb is seen. Abnormalities inside the womb such as polyps, fibroids, cancer and infectious changes can then be detected. With the patient under general anaesthesia and lying down with her legs supported, the hysteroscope is gently inserted through the vagina into the cervix to gain access to the inner surface of the womb. The hysteroscope can also be used to remove polyps and fibroids of the womb as well as to destroy an abnormally thick lining which is a common cause for excessive vaginal bleeding.

Q What is falloposcopy?

A In falloposcopy, the falloposcope is passed through the lower portion of the uterus upwards to where the Fallopian tube enters the womb. This procedure allows the inner opening of the Fallopian tube to be examined and is carried out primarily in fertility investigations. As in hysteroscopy, the patient is placed under a short general anaesthesia.

Q What is cystoscopy?

A Cystoscopy is the examination of the cavity of the bladder using an instrument called the cystoscope. This can be done in the clinic as an outpatient procedure as no anaesthesia is required. The cystoscope is inserted into the urethra and the inner surface examined. In this manner, small stones in the bladder and polyps can be seen and removed or cancer diagnosed. Another very important use of this procedure is in the investigation of urge incontinence arising from instability of the bladder muscles. Through the cystoscope, increasing amounts of saline is pumped into the bladder and the internal pressure constantly monitored. The muscles of the bladder wall are said to be 'irritable' when the patient feels like passing urine and when contractions of the bladder muscles occur at lower filling volumes of the bladder than normal.

Q What is laparoscopy?

A This is an extremely popular procedure which has widespread applications in gynaecology. The uses of laparoscopy can be divided into two groups, namely, diagnostic laparoscopy and therapeutic laparoscopy.

Q What is diagnostic laparoscopy?

A This is the use of laparoscopy to find out the various causes of the ailment. Indications for diagnostic laparoscopy include:

1. Cases of infertility, when the procedure is carried out to detect endometriosis and blockage of the Fallopian tubes
2. Establishing the cause of pain in the lower abdomen over a long period (chronic pelvic pain)
3. Establishing the presence of a pregnancy outside the womb, for example in the Fallopian tube (ectopic pregnancy)
4. The follow-up of patients after treatment for ovarian cancer in order to detect early recurrence

Q What is therapeutic laparoscopy?

A These are procedures in which the laparoscope is used to actually treat disease. Examples include:

1. Removal of ovarian cysts (ovarian cystectomy)
2. Removal of fibroids of the womb (myomectomy)
3. Destroying endometriosis using laser (laser vaporization)
4. Removing an ectopic pregnancy and at the same time preserving the tube (salpingostomy)

5. Freeing the Fallopian tubes when infertility is caused by scar tissue from endometriosis or previous infection (salpingolysis or adhesiolysis)

6. Transferring the sperm-and-egg mixture into the outer end of the Fallopian tube in GIFT procedures for infertility

7. Sterilization procedures for women who do not want to have any more children

8. Removal of intrauterine contraceptive devices which have moved out of the uterine cavity

9. Bringing forward a womb which is tilted backwards (retroverted uterus)

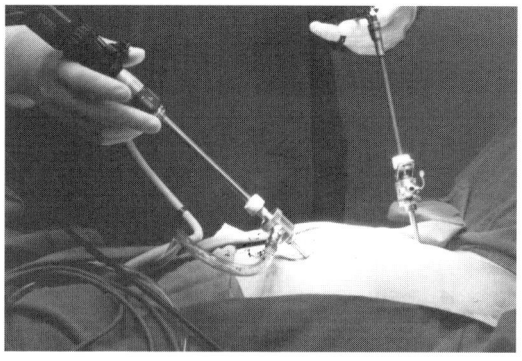

In laparoscopy, the viewing laparoscope on the left allows the surgeon to look at the inside of the body on a TV screen. The instrument for removing the cyst is on the right.

Q   What are the possible complications with the various 'scopies'?

A   Colposcopy is a safe procedure with no complications except that abnormal changes in the cervix can be easily missed by a gynaecologist who is not trained in this special field. There is a small risk of perforation of the uterus if hysteroscopy or fallopscopy is performed by an inexperienced surgeon.

As for laparoscopy, complications can be divided into those associated with general anaesthesia and those as a result of the procedure itself. In addition to the usual anaesthetic risks, there is the possibility of irregular heart rhythms and even heart attacks occurring if the carbon dioxide gas is pumped too rapidly into the abdominal cavity during the procedure. Complications due to the procedure itself include injuries to the bowel and major internal blood vessels, bleeding and infection of the internal lining of the pelvic cavity (peritonitis). Injuries to the bowel and other organs are more common in the presence of extensive scar tissue (adhesions) or with less than careful use of the laser.

Q With these possible complications, why would anyone want to go for laparoscopic surgery?

A Firstly, these complications are uncommon. Secondly, pain is much less during the postoperative period when compared to conventional surgery. For example, the laparoscopic removal of a 5-cm ovarian cyst results in the patient nursing 3 tiny wounds measuring between 0.5 and 1 cm on the abdominal surface postoperatively. This causes much less pain than the usual incision which averages 5-cm. Thirdly, the patient can often go home the very same day compared to a 4- to 5- day hospital stay for conventional surgery. Fourthly, as a result of the shorter hospital stay, the possible heart attack on seeing the hospital bill is avoided!

Lastly, the optics of the laparoscope allows a better view of certain awkward nooks and crannies within the abdominal cavity. These can at best be viewed with great difficulty with the naked eye in conventional surgery. Examples of this include the detection of tumour recurrence on the upper back portion of the liver when laparoscopy is performed following treatment for cancer of the ovary.

Q Are there any patients who should not undergo laparoscopy?

A Laparoscopy should not be performed on patients with infection of the pelvic cavity (peritonitis), swelling of the bowel following obstruction and large ovarian cysts when there is suspicion of cancer. This is because to remove a large cyst through a small surgical opening the surgeon would have to puncture the cyst first, which will theoretically lead to the spread of the cancer cells. Laparoscopy should also not be offered to patients with severe heart or lung disease as the inflation of the abdomen with carbon dioxide gas may compromise the function of these organs further. Lastly, laparoscopy should not be done on a patient pregnant beyond 14 weeks.

The common procedures that a woman may undergo can be conveniently classified into a few broad groups: simple out-patient procedures, some of which require local anaesthesia, minor surgery requiring short general anaesthesia and major surgery.

Simple out-patient procedures

Simple procedures that are done in the clinic with the patient fully awake

The Pap smear
Colposcopy
High vaginal swabs
Postcoital test

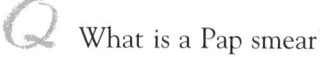

What is a Pap smear?

The Pap smear, named after the Greek physician G. N. Papanicolaou, is a simple procedure used to detect cancer of the cervix. The advantage of the Pap smear is that it is a simple painless procedure causing minimal discomfort to the patient. The doctor uses a wooden spoon to scrape the surface of the cervix, thereby obtaining cells. The cells are placed on a glass slide and examined by the cytologist. In this way, abnormal or cancerous cells are detected. The disadvantage of the Pap smear is that it is only about 95 per cent accurate in detecting disease because sometimes, a small area of cancer may be missed in the scraping procedure.

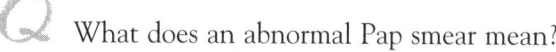

What does an abnormal Pap smear mean?

This is a result which sends waves of panic through most women. In actual fact, there is often not much to worry about. The results of the smear are classified into five groups, namely:

A class one smear means the cells are normal.

A class two smear indicates infection of the cervix.

A class three smear suggests precancerous change of the cervix.

A class four smear is highly suggestive of cancer of the cervix.

A class five smear means that obvious cancer cells are seen.

An abnormal Pap smear is therefore a result other than class one but it is only in classes four and five where there exists an obvious threat to life. Fortunately these classes of Pap smear are not common.

Q Why is it necessary to go for routine Pap smears?

A It is very wise to go for routine Pap smears as cancer of the cervix usually develops over a long time and progresses from precancer (mild, moderate and then severe dysplasia) to cancer. Regular Pap smears enable the disease to be detected at the early precancerous stage and this is very easily and painlessly treated by freezing the cervix (cryosurgery) or burning the cervix (laser vaporization). Also, the cervix is an accessible part of the woman's body, unlike the ovary which is an internal organ, and hence detecting disease is relatively simple.

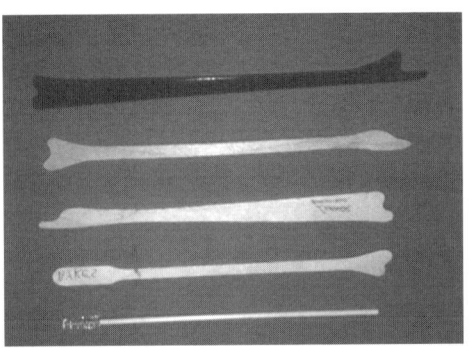

Instruments used for Pap smears

Q What needs to be done when there is an abnormal Pap smear?

A The next step is to confirm the diagnosis. The gynaecologist will perform a colposcopy and if necessary remove a small piece of tissue for examination (punch biopsy). Colposcopy is an essential complement to the Pap smear in the detection of precancer or early cancer of the cervix as it can detect very small areas of abnormal change.

Q What is a high vaginal swab?

A This is a painless procedure that is carried out when a patient complains of increased vaginal discharge, abnormal discharge with an offensive smell or colour or itchiness of the vulva. Using a small cotton bud, discharge from the vagina is taken and sent to the laboratory. In this way, infections with *Candida* or *Trichomonas*, or other diseases can be detected and the appropriate treatment given.

Simple out-patient procedures with local anaesthesia

Simple procedures that are done in the clinic with the patient awake but with a teeny bit of local anaesthesia

Excision of simple lumps and bumps
Endometrial sampling

Sometimes, a woman wakes up in the morning, looks into the mirror and finds the beautiful contours of her face marred by a lump which was not there before. Or she may, on taking a bath, find a bump on her body.

Q What are common lumps which may occur on the face?

A A common lump which occurs on the face is the dermoid cyst, which is usually noticed over the forehead, root of the nose or the outer part of the eyelid. It contains fluid and hence feels firm to the touch.

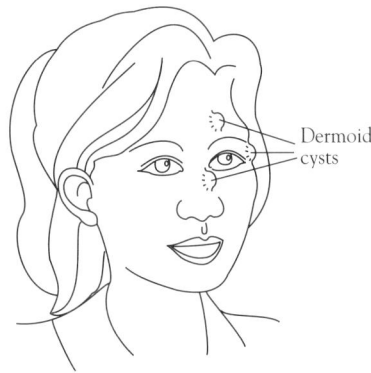

These are the likely spots for dermoid cysts.

Q What other cysts are commonly seen?

A Another cyst which occurs quite commonly is the sebaceous cyst. This has a smooth, rounded appearance and contains oily material. These cysts can be found anywhere over the body and are usually painless unless complicated by infection.

Q Apart from cysts, are there any other common lumps?

A Another common lump is the lipoma. This is a non-cancerous collection of fat cells and is usually found on the shoulders or back but can occur anywhere on the body.

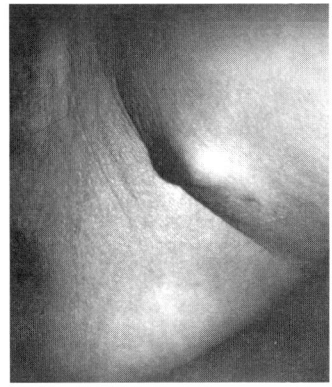

A lipoma on the inside of the upper thigh

Q Is there a simple way to differentiate a lipoma from a sebaceous cyst?

A A cyst usually contains fluid whereas the lipoma does not. When a strong pencil torch light is placed over the bump, a cyst will 'light up' (transilluminate) whereas a lipoma will not.

Q How are these lumps treated?

A Small dermoid cysts, sebaceous cysts or lipomas found on the body, arms or legs can be easily removed in the clinic under local anaesthesia. The patient is placed in a position which exposes the cyst and an injection of local anaesthetic given under the skin. Once numbness has set in, the surgeon makes a tiny cut over the cyst and uses a pair of forceps to tease out the wall of the cyst or lipoma. Any bleeding is then stopped by using stitches and the surface of the cut closed with sutures. A dressing is then placed over the wound and the patient sent home.

Q What is a papilloma?

A This is a nipple-like growth on the surface of the skin. It is benign and is easily removed with a simple cut under local anaesthesia. The cut is then stitched up and the patient goes home the same day.

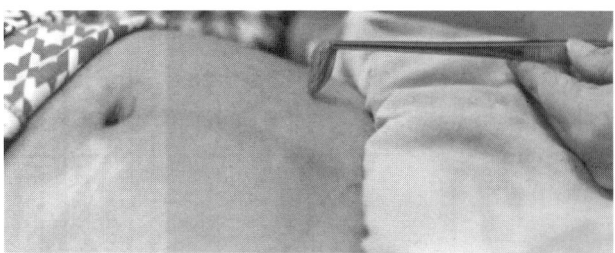

A papilloma of the abdominal wall

Minor procedures with short general anaesthesia

Minor procedures done in the operating theatre with a short anaesthesia

D & C
Removal of Bartholin's cyst
Removal of a breast lump

Q I am 40 years old and am having irregular bleeding. My general practitioner feels that I should have a D & C. What is a D & C?

A D & C stands for dilatation and curettage. In essence, it means dilating the cervix and then using a metal spoon-like instrument (curette) to scrape the inner surface of the womb.

Q When is it necessary to do a D & C?

A A D & C is usually performed for abnormal vaginal bleeding. Before the age of 40 years, abnormal bleeding is usually the result of a hormonal imbalance and can be treated by drugs alone. If the bleeding is still very heavy or continues despite treatment with medication, then a D & C may be necessary to arrest the bleeding.

After the age of 40 years and especially after the menopause, irregular abnormal bleeding may have a more serious cause, for example cancer of the womb. In such a case, there is a stronger reason to perform a D & C so that the tissue removed can be sent to the laboratory for examination. This is the same as the procedure performed after a miscarriage to remove pieces of placenta left behind as these will otherwise cause an infection.

Q Are there any possible complications in doing a D & C?

A A D & C is generally very safe. However, complications are still possible. These include injuries to the cervix and the body of the womb. The latter occurs when the metal instrument used to dilate the cervix is pushed through the wall of the womb (perforation) and this can lead to a significant amount of bleeding. Later complications may arise from damage to the cervix and these include miscarriages in subsequent pregnancies. Following a D & C, the surface of the womb is raw and bacteria may settle in to cause an infection.

Q What is a Bartholin's cyst?

A A Bartholin's cyst is a swelling of the Bartholin's gland, which is situated over the lower third of the vulva. It has an opening at the junction of the vagina and the vulva.

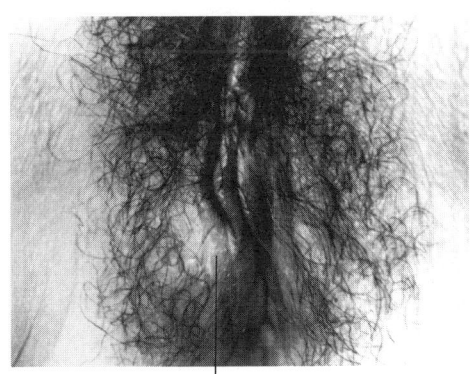

A Bartholin's cyst

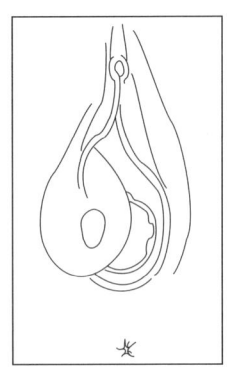

A Bartholin's cyst

This cyst often becomes infected to form an abscess which is acutely painful and tender. In fact, a Bartholin's abscess is a condition which I can often diagnose just by looking at how my patient walks and sits. She would be sitting on the edge of the chair and putting her weight on the unaffected side.

Q How is a Bartholin's cyst treated?

A With the patient under a short general anaesthesia, the surface of the cyst is cut with a sharp scalpel and the fluid drained. The edges of the cyst are then stitched together. The cavity is packed with a thin gauze soaked in antiseptic solution which is removed only after 3 days. This prevents closure of the opening of the gland and recurrent cyst formation. Here is a first-person account:

I woke up one morning feeling as though there was a piece of hot charcoal in my vagina. It was so painful that I could not put my legs together. Driving to the clinic was pure agony and I suffered even worse agony when I was examined. My gynaecologist diagnosed the condition as an infected Bartholin's cyst and advised immediate surgery. I'm actually very squeamish but I actually looked forward to the surgery on account of the pain.

In the operating theatre, the anaesthetist gave me an injection on my left hand and I blacked out. When I awoke, the difference was incredible! The pain had completely gone and I could see and hear birds chirping outside my window.

Q I felt a lump in my left breast today. I'm worried sick. What should I do?

A The first thing to do is not to worry. Breast lumps are common and 90 per cent of them are benign. You should see your doctor, who will determine whether the lump is cystic or solid. In the former case, a fine needle will be used to suck out the fluid and this will settle the problem. If the lump is solid, then surgery to remove it is advisable.

Q What are the signs that the lump is cancerous?

A A cancerous lump is usually hard and fixed to the skin whereas a benign lump is usually firm and mobile. Also, the skin above a cancerous lump may be dimpled, so that the skin appears like that of an orange. A patient with a cancerous lump may also have swellings in the armpits which are enlarged lymph nodes.

Q Is the surgery painful? Will I have a scar?

A The surgery itself is hardly painful as it will be performed under anaesthesia. Following the surgery, there will be some discomfort for a few days. There will also be minimal scarring as most of the time the cut is made at the junction of the dark skin of the areola and the fairer skin of the rest of the breast. A very fine suture is also used and when this is removed, only a thin fine line is seen.

Q What is a frozen section?

A When a frozen section is done, the tissue removed is first frozen in liquid nitrogen and then examined immediately. The pathologist makes an immediate diagnosis. With the patient still under anaesthesia, more extensive surgery can be carried out if the lump is cancerous and the patient need not be subjected to a second operation. Otherwise, the usual pathological diagnosis involves staining the tissue with paraffin and it takes a few days before the results are available. Here is a first-person account:

I was taking a bath last week when I felt a hard lump on the underside of my left breast. I felt it again and I broke out in cold sweat! It was like a little peanut under the skin. I was terrified. Cancer came to my mind. I've just been married and my husband loves the look and feel of my breasts. How can I face him if I have to lose a breast?

The words of reassurance from my gynaecologist did not help. I agreed to have the lump removed and examined immediately under what he called a frozen section. I was thinking of suicide if it was cancer. I was too depressed to feel anything as they pushed me into the operating room. I felt an injection and I blacked out.

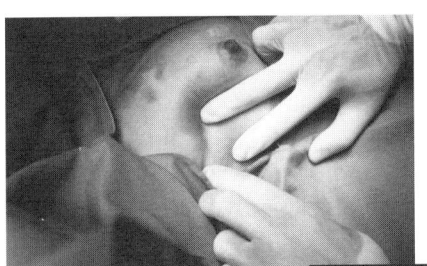

First, the surgeon locates the lump.

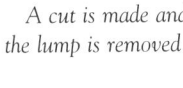

A cut is made and the lump is removed.

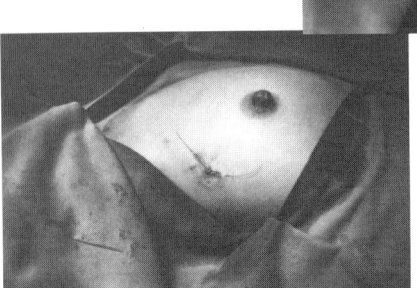

The cut is then stitched together.

When I woke up, my left breast ached and I could not lift my arm. I saw some roses on the table and a little note from my husband saying that he would love me no matter what happened. I cried. I looked at my chest and saw a large plaster below the nipple At least the breast was still there! My gynaecologist soon came in and told me that the lump was found to be benign. I felt an enormous weight roll of my chest. That same evening, I went home thanking God for his mercy and for a wonderful husband.

Five days later, I returned to the clinic to have the stitch taken out. It itched a bit but it was painless. I could hardly see any scar and am really very happy.

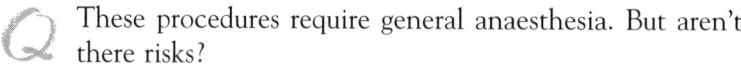

Major procedures

Major procedures done in the operating with a general anaesthesia

Cone biopsy of the cervix
Removal of an ovarian cyst (ovarian cystectomy)
Removal of fibroids of the womb (myomectomy)
Removal of the womb (hysterectomy)
Removal of the vulva (vulvectomy)
Pelvic floor repair
Microsurgery for blocked tubes

Q These procedures require general anaesthesia. But aren't there risks?

A Firstly, complications are extremely uncommon. Possible complications include a fall in the oxygen level in the blood, irregular heartbeats and a fall in blood pressure during the operation.

For a few days after the operation, the patient may have a sore throat, headache, dizziness and nausea but these sumptoms soon disappear.

Cone biopsy of the cervix

Q What is a cone biopsy of the cervix?

A A cone biopsy of the cervix is a procedure in which a cone-shaped piece of tissue the size of the tip of one's nose is removed from the neck of the womb.

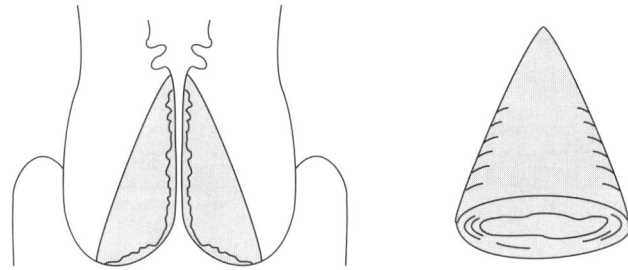

In a cone biopsy, the shaded part of the cervix is removed.

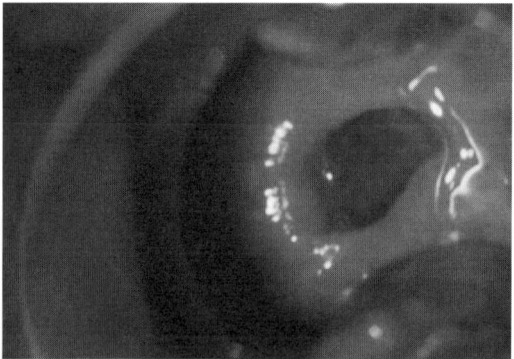

A cervix after a cone biopsy, as seen through a speculum.

This is usually done as treatment for precancer of the cervix where the removal of the whole diseased portion is enough to bring about a cure. Sometimes when the cone biopsy is examined, it is found that actual cancer has developed. The depth of malignant penetration can then be determined and this is essential in deciding the best form of treatment for the cancer. In some cases, removal of the whole uterus is sufficient whereas in others additional treatment like radiotherapy or chemotherapy would be necessary.

Q Is a cone biopsy painful?

A Surprisingly, this procedure is not painful as the cervix does not have the usual nerve fibres that the vulva has. A light anaesthesia is all that is required and there is no postoperative pain.

Q What are the possible complications of a cone biopsy?

A The most common complication of a cone biopsy is bleeding during and immediately after the operation. Using the latest techniques like the laser or the electromagnetic instrument, bleeding is minimized as open blood vessels can be sealed off immediately. Infection can also complicate the surgery when bacteria colonizes the raw surface of the cervix and this results in bleeding a week to 10 days later (secondary haemorrhage). Late complications of cone biopsy include late miscarriages due to damage to the neck of the womb.

Removal of ovarian cysts

Q What is an ovarian cyst? Is it different from a fibroid?

A An ovarian cyst is a fluid-filled structure, similar to a small water-filled balloon, arising from one or both ovaries.

A cyst is different from a fibroid in that it stems from the ovary whereas a fibroid arises from the uterus. Also, a fibroid is solid as it is made of muscle fibres, unlike a cyst which contains fluid. From the medical point of view, an ovarian cyst is more ominous as it has a 5 per cent chance of being cancerous. A fibroid is only very rarely malignant.

Q Are there different types of ovarian cyst?

A Ovarian cysts comes in different sizes and types. About 95 per cent of ovarian cysts are non-cancerous and these can be broadly classified into five groups:

1. Functional cysts. These arise from changes in the ovaries as a result of ovulation or hormonal imbalances. These cysts are only temporary.
2. Endometriotic cysts. These cysts contain blood which may become thick and brown (chocolate cysts). There is a strong association between endometriotic cysts and infertility.
3. Cysts containing mucus (mucinous cystadenoma). These account for 15 per cent of benign ovarian cysts and are usually found only in one ovary.
4. Cysts containing clear fluid (serous cystadenoma). These are more serious than the mucus-containing variety and account for 23 per cent of benign ovarian cysts. It is found in both ovaries in 15 per cent of patients.

5. Dermoid cysts. These are interesting cysts which contain oily, greasy material mixed with hair, bone and occasionally a tooth! It is heavy and has a tendency to become twisted (torsion of ovarian cyst).

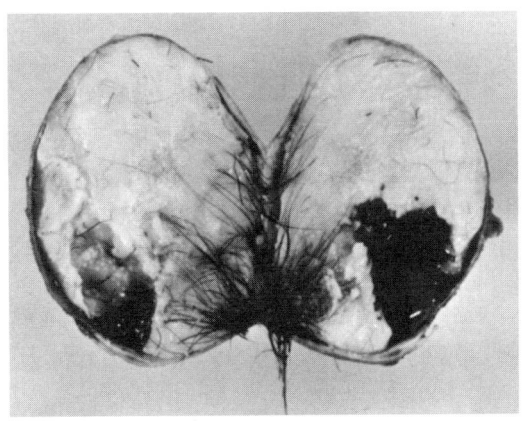

A dermoid cyst cut in half

Q   What are the symptoms of an ovarian cyst?

A   Although there are many different types of ovarian cyst, they usually give rise to similar problems. The woman usually complains of pain or discomfort on one side of the lower abdomen. This is commonly described as a dull ache, twinge or a feeling of heaviness. Pain becomes intense and unremitting if the whole ovary together with the cyst becomes twisted (torsion). As the cyst enlarges and presses on adjacent organs, the patient may complain of constipation or the frequent desire to pass urine. Pain on intercourse especially on deep penetration is another symptom.

As the ovary is an internal organ, it is quite common for the cyst to be symptomless until it has grown to a large size. In this instance, the patient complains of progressive enlargement of the lower abdomen. I had a patient come to see me after the New Year when she found that she could not get into her *cheong-sam*. On examination, she was found to have a left ovarian cyst the size of a water-melon, which was totally painless.

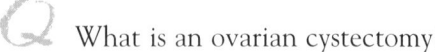

I have an ovarian cyst. Should I have it removed?

This is a vexing question. The decision mainly hinges on the possibility of cancer. Cysts which are found on both ovaries or recurrent cysts are more likely to be malignant. An ultrasound scan would aid in the diagnosis as malignant cysts tend to have solid areas and contain partitions (septa) whereas benign cysts tend not to. Also, measurement of blood flow to malignant cysts would reveal an increased rate of flow as these cysts have a higher rate of growth.

Bearing in mind that small benign-looking cysts can have small areas of malignant change, the final diagnosis can only be made with the specimen removed and examined by the pathologist. Hence, any cyst which has a possibility of being malignant should be removed because ovarian cancer is a highly dangerous disease. This is because it is often silent and therefore treatment usually commences only at a late stage. Early diagnosis is therefore crucial for the patient's long-term survival.

What is an ovarian cystectomy?

This is an operation to remove the cyst in the ovary and then repair the rest of the ovary. This is performed when the cyst is benign and healthy ovarian tissue is present. In some instances, the ovarian cyst grows to such an extent that the whole ovary is destroyed. In such patients, the whole ovary and the cyst is removed (oophorectomy). This is also performed when there is a suspicion of malignancy at the time of the operation.

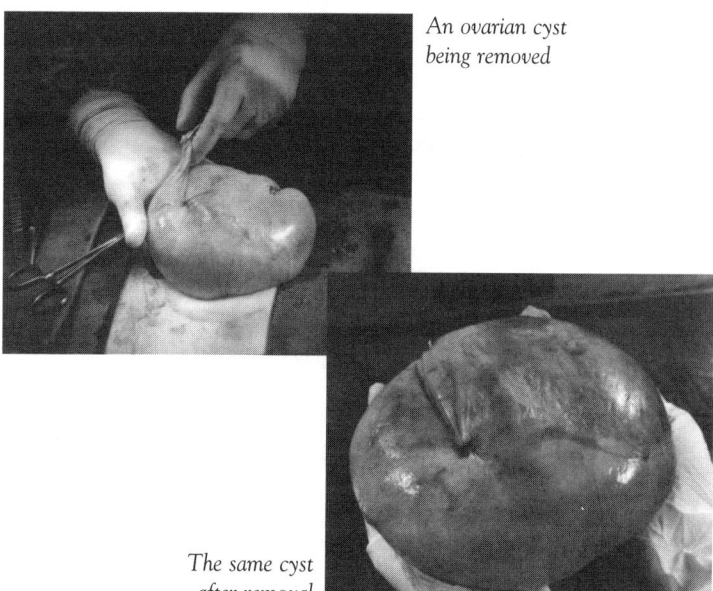

An ovarian cyst being removed

The same cyst after removal

Q How can this be done? Is it painful?

A An ovarian cystectomy is major surgery and is performed either using the laparoscope or through a cut of 4 to 7 cm above the pubic hair line. The laparoscope is chosen if the cyst is not too large and has no features of malignancy. The operation is performed under general anaesthesia and hence the operation itself is painless. After the surgery, the patient is given pain-killers through an intravenous drip. Usually, no food or fluid is given for 24 hours. The following day, fluids are given orally and the patient is given tablets of pain-killers once the drip is removed. As such, the patient hardly feels any pain except for a dull ache over the operation wound when she moves.

Removal of fibroids of the womb

Q What is a fibroid?

A A uterine fibroid is the commonest non-malignant tumour in the human body. It is made up of smooth muscle fibres and, like the ovarian cyst, can grow to horrendous sizes. Unlike the ovarian cyst, the uterine fibroid is rarely malignant.

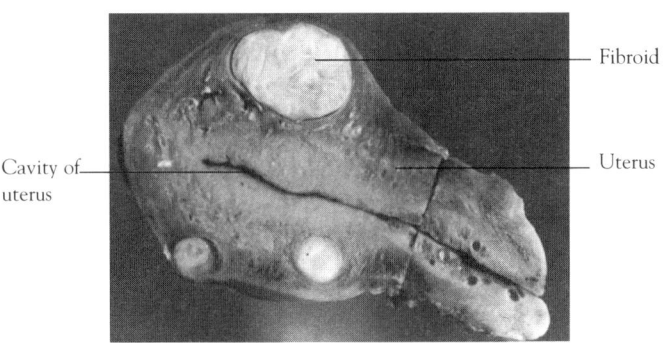

Fibroid

Cavity of uterus

Uterus

This uterus has been cut in half. Note the three white growths in the wall of the uterus. These are fibroids.

Q What are the causes of a uterine fibroid?

A A hormonal imbalance with a higher level of oestrogen influence is believed to be a factor in the formation of fibroids but the actual cause is not clearly known. Fibroids tend to occur in women in the higher socio-economic classes, like the busy executive who puts off childbearing until a late age. In fact, women who have given birth to many children tend to have a lower incidence of fibroids. Some gynaecologists sum up the situation dramatically: 'The womb, after waiting for years and years to produce a baby, gets so frustrated that it decides to produce fibroids instead!'

Q What does a woman complain of if she has a fibroid?

A Fibroids may be completely silent or there may be symptoms related to their position or their size. In the former case, fibroids which enlarge the inner lining of the womb (a) would cause heavy menstrual bleeding and those which protrude out of the cavity (polyps) (b) may cause a cramping pain, especially during the menses as the womb contracts and tries to expel the fibroid.

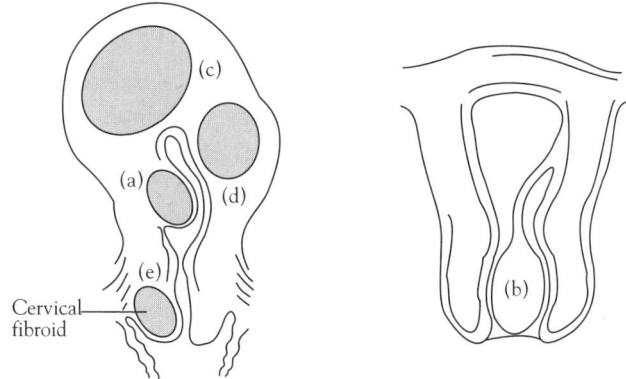

Uterine fibroids can be found in any of these positions.

Fibroids located at the front of the womb would press on the bladder and cause the patient to feel like passing urine often whereas those situated at the back (c) would press on the rectum and give the feeling of incomplete emptying of the bowel. Fibroids which compress the Fallopian tube where it enters the womb (cornual fibroids) (d) will cause infertility because of tubal blockage.

Fibroids can also cause problems related to their size. In very large fibroids, the patient would notice swelling of the abdomen. A large fibroid situated over the lower portion of the womb (e) would affect the position of the baby, leading to a breech presentation. It could also interfere with the dilatation of the cervix during labour, so that a Caesarean section would be necessary.

Q I have a fibroid. Do I need an operation?

A I personally have less compunction to remove a fibroid than an ovarian cyst as fibroids are rarely malignant. Whether or not you need surgery depends on whether the fibroid is troubling you, for example, causing heavy menstruation to the point of anaemia or preventing conception by causing blockage of the Fallopian tubes. By virtue of their size, fibroids which cause the womb to be larger than as if it was at the 12th week of pregnancy should be removed. This is because at this size, the fibroid would eventually cause problems. If done at a later stage, it would pose a higher operative risk as the patient would be older and more likely to suffer from medical complications like high blood pressure or heart disease.

Q Are there different operations to remove fibroids?

A The operation to remove fibroids is known as a myomectomy. Depending on the size of the fibroid, this can be done either via the laparoscope or through the usual method of a horizontal cut of 5 to 10 cm just above the pubic hair line. Fibroids located over the cervix can also be removed from the vagina.

At the time of the operation, the fibroid is shelled out, rather like taking the egg yolk out from the egg white in a hard-boiled egg. This leaves a cavity which must be securely stitched up as bleeding from open blood vessels can be torrential. If there is a likelihood of further bleeding later on, the surgeon will usually leave a 'drain' in place. This is a plastic tube which looks quite frightening to the patient or her relatives as it comes right out of the skin into a vacuum bottle which collects the stale blood. The drain actually does not cause any pain at all. After a day or so when the bleeding subsides and no more blood enters the bottle, the drain is removed. Here is a first-person account of a myomectomy:

For a long time, I had felt under the weather, although I could not put my finger on the cause. Upon advice, I decided to consult a gynaecologist.

At the clinic, I was told to drink lots of water. When my bladder was uncomfortably full, I went in to see the gynaecologist. He asked me a whole lot of questions and then carried out an ultrasound scan. He placed a device like a computer mouse on my lower abdomen and a fan-shaped image appeared on a screen above us. We saw the culprit – a roundish lump – which he said was a fibroid and which he said had to come out.

The day for the surgery came. As I settled into my hospital bed, my eyes strayed over to some strange things on the table at the foot of the bed. These were for my enema, the smiling nurse said. She told me to lie on my side while she introduced a fluid into my bowels through a tube-like instrument. It made my insides uncomfortable but it helped that the nurse explained what she was doing at every stage. I held in the fluid for as long as I could. Some minutes and four visits to the toilet later, I was really clean. Next, the nurse shaved my pubic area. I kept still, so there were no cuts.

Soon I was wheeled into the operating theatre. There the anaesthetist explained how he would put me to sleep. Attentive nurses told me of the machines they hooked me up to and of what use they were. I humoured them good-naturedly and acted suitably impressed. But soon I felt drowsy so I shut my eyes for a moment. When I opened them, the operation was over.

I was wheeled back to my room. They lifted me off the trolley and began to slide me into my bed. I called out to them to take care, or I tried to, but no words came out. I spent the next few hours alternating between chatting with my visitors and drifting off to sleep.

When I became more alert later that night, I realized, to my relief, that the wound did not hurt much. It was just extremely uncomfortable. I also realized that a catheter was in place to drain the urine. Two days later, they removed it. Soon I was able to get out of bed and walk carefully to the toilet by myself. After passing wind (Now, that hurt!) and moving my bowels, I was ready to go home.

Ten days later, I had my stitches removed. I did not even skip a period, although the first one after the surgery was very painful. I was back at my normal activities some months later. It has been a year and a half after my operation and I have never felt better!

What are the dangers of myomectomies?

A myomectomy is actually a very safe procedure even though it is a major operation with the attendant risks of a general anaesthesia. Other possible dangers are bleeding at the time of operation, with possible infection in the pelvis if stale blood is not removed at the time of surgery or via a drain later on. If the fibroid removed involves the inner surface of the womb, then there is weakening of the wall of the womb with the theoretical possibility of rupture of the womb in subsequent pregnancies. In this instance, a Caesarean section should be performed 2 weeks before the expected date of delivery.

Q Are there any drugs which can shrink fibroids?

A There is a drug which is a GnRH analogue which has been shown in clinical trials to cause a reduction in size for 90 per cent of fibroids. Those that do not respond are usually calcified. Of those that shrink, there is a reduction of 50 to 70 per cent in size and this occurs after 4 to 6 months of treatment.

Q Are there any side-effects to this treatment?

A Some women experience hot flushes, irregular bleeding or spotting, dryness of the vagina or pain during intercourse. Prolonged treatment may lead to thinning of the bones but patients normally recover from this 8 months after stopping treatment.

Removal of the womb

Q What is a hysterectomy?

A A hysterectomy is an operation to remove the whole womb. It is aptly named because many women are close to hysteria at the prospect of losing their wombs! In actual fact, the prefix 'hyster' refers to the womb.

Q What are the situations in which the uterus needs to be removed?

A Conditions which require a hysterectomy are numerous. They can be conveniently divided into non-cancerous conditions and those due to malignancy. Benign diseases for which a hysterectomy is indicated include heavy bleeding causing anaemia or severe crippling pain during menstruation poorly controlled by medication, multiple uterine fibroids distorting the whole uterus and prolapse of the uterus.

A hysterectomy is usually performed in the older patient not desirous of fertility as the removal of the womb obviously makes further childbearing impossible. There are occasions in which the womb is removed even though it is healthy, for example, in a 50-year-old woman who is having surgery for bilateral ovarian cysts. In this instance, there is little reason to retain the uterus as childbearing is no longer an issue and the removal of the uterus frees the patient from the risk of developing a disease such as cancer of the cervix later on.

Malignant conditions for which a hysterectomy need to be performed include cancer of the womb or ovaries, early stages of cancer of the cervix or cancer of the Fallopian tubes, the last of which is a rare condition.

Q I am 45 years old and need to have my womb removed because of fibroids. Should I remove the ovaries as well?

A This depends very much on the state of the ovaries at the time of surgery. Healthy ovaries should be retained as they serve a vital function in producing the hormones oestrogen and progesterone. These play an important role in delaying the onset of hot flushes, heart disease and osteoporosis. On the other hand, ovaries which appear small and 'burnt out' or diseased ovaries should be removed at the time of surgery as these have limited use and are sources of potential disease in the future.

Q What about removing the appendix at the time of hysterectomy?

A The appendix is a functionless organ in the human being and can cause problems if it becomes inflamed (acute appendicitis). Removal of the appendix (appendicectomy) at the time of a hysterectomy, although convenient, increases the risk of complications, especially postoperative fever and infection. This is because an appendicectomy allows the bacteria from the colon access to the raw hysterectomy site and this may lead to serious infections (peritonitis). I would advise an appendicectomy only if the appendix is easily accessible, as well as long and tortuous. These appendices have a higher chance of getting infected in the future.

I remember a 48-year-old patient who was scheduled for a hysterectomy for a large uterine fibroid and who also wanted her appendix taken out at the same time as her sister had had appendicitis a week before. I was very reluctant to do so but she was adamant. At the time of surgery, there was minimal blood loss, the raw edges of the hysterectomy were well covered and the appendix was easily accessible. I performed the appendicectomy at the time of the hysterectomy and sent the tissue for examination. Imagine my surprise when the results showed early cancer of the appendix, a very, very rare condition! Now every time I see her, this dear patient never fails to give me the 'I told you so' look.

Q How many ways can a hysterectomy be done?

A A hysterectomy can be performed either through the vagina or through a cut in the abdomen. In vaginal hysterectomy, the whole uterus is removed through the vagina and this is usually performed together with tightening of the vagina (pelvic floor repair) when there is descent of the womb. One way to do this is through the vagina solely, where there will be no cuts in the abdomen. It can also be done with the aid of a laparoscope (laparoscopically-assisted vaginal hysterectomy), where there will be three additional puncture wounds on the surface of the abdomen.

In an abdominal hysterectomy, a horizontal cut 6 to 8 cm long is made on the surface of the abdomen just above the pubic hair line and the uterus removed through this incision.

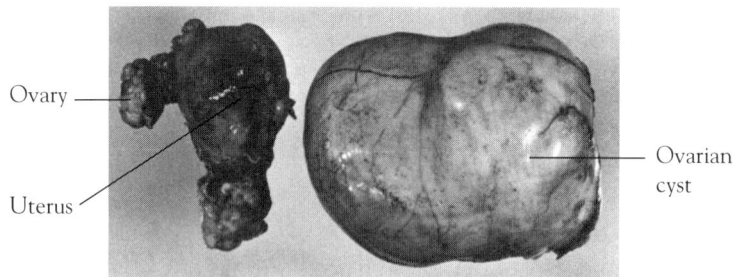

A uterus, an ovary and an ovarian cyst removed surgically. Notice the size of the cyst.

What are the possible complications of a hysterectomy?

A hysterectomy is a relatively safe procedure with a mortality rate of 0.2 per 1000 cases. Apart from anaesthetic complications, there could be bleeding at the time of the operation or injuries to adjacent organs like the ureter (the tube-like structure which allows urine to pass from the kidney to the bladder) or intestines. This can occur when there are extensive adhesions (scar tissue) which forms as a result of past pelvic infection or endometriosis.

Later complications include vaginal dryness as the cervix is no longer there to contribute to vaginal discharge. Psychological effects include depression and the feeling of a lack of femininity. Here is a first-person account of a patient with cancer of the cervix:

Cancer only happens to someone else, never yourself, I believed. Then one day after sex, I noticed a pink stain on my panties. Over the next few days, it persisted. I was worried. I had not stepped into any clinic for the past 5 years and was genuinely terrified. My worst fears were confirmed when the gynaecologist examined me. I could see my own cervix with this instrument he used and there was a large ugly growth with some blood coming from it. The diagnosis of cancer was confirmed after a piece of the tissue was examined.

My whole life flashed past me. I have lived my life pretty much the way I wanted and life has been good to me. I am strong, attractive and independent. But now, for the first time in my 35 years, I felt truly vulnerable. My gynaecologist gave me two options, radiotherapy or surgery. He advised surgery as my cancer was at what he called stage one. The advantages, he said, were that my ovaries would be preserved and that I would still be able to have a normal sex life. I agreed and went through a whole battery of tests before they admitted me for the surgery.

That morning, they wheeled me to the theatre and gave me an injection. I felt light headed and before I knew it, someone was calling my name and telling me to wake up. I felt a little pain on my tummy. I was back in the ward and I had two tubes sticking out from me. After a few days, they removed the tubes. My gynaecologist told me that the cancer had not spread any further and that I have an 85 per cent chance of a cure. I guess it is good to be an optimist and not brood over the other 15 per cent. I was discharged after one week.

For the next two weeks I had trouble passing urine and was always constipated. My gynaecologist told me that this was temporary as the nerves of the pelvis were slightly damaged because of the extensive operation but that I would eventually recover. He then prescribed some laxatives. Over the next 2 months, I got better.

I am looking forward to my new lease of life. I have always been a fighter and will definitely not let this disease get me down. I have thrown away all my cigarettes, lighters and ashtrays.

Pelvic floor repair

Q What is a pelvic floor repair?

A A pelvic floor repair is, in essence, the removal of loose vaginal skin and tightening of the muscles and tissues of the vagina. It may involve only the front (anterior repair) which usually involves a Kelly's stitch to correct stress incontinence or the back (posterior colpoperineorrhaphy), or both.

Q What are the conditions which warrant a pelvic floor repair?

A An anterior repair with a Kelly's stitch is usually performed for troublesome stress incontinence or the feeling of incomplete emptying of the bladder due to a large cystocele. A posterior repair is often carried out at the same time if the posterior wall of the vagina is lax, with bulging of the intestines above (enterocele) or of the rectum below (rectocele).

Sometimes, a pelvic floor repair is requested for sexual problems. This occurs when a loose vagina results in a lack of sexual stimulation or orgasm failure in the woman or her partner. Just the other day, I had two middle-aged women who were neighbours come to see me for a pelvic floor repair. For months, both their husbands would go off for overnight trips. They had just discovered sadly that the so-called fishing trips were actually sexual trysts with their younger mistresses.

Microsurgery for blocked tubes

Q What is microsurgery?

A Microsurgery is the surgical technique which involves the use of the operating microscope and very fine surgical instruments in very delicate repair procedures. Sutures used in microsurgery are thinner than the human hair.

Q When is microsurgery required?

A Microsurgical techniques are usually required in the treatment of infertility. For example, the Fallopian tubes may be blocked at the ends from adhesions caused by endometriosis or past pelvic infection. In such a case, the operating microscope is needed for the very delicate freeing of the ends of the Fallopian tubes. Sometimes, a portion of the Fallopian tube would be blocked either from past infection or from a previous sterilization operation. The blocked portion of the tube is then cut and the two ends joined again using microsurgical techniques. This involves having to put 16 stitches (2 rows of 8 stitches) in a tube only 4 mm in diameter such that a canal of 1 mm is left open at the end of the operation! The guiding principle in microsurgery is minimal tissue damage with minimal bleeding so that there is good healing and the restoration of the normal anatomy and function of the tubes.

Q Is microsurgery painful?

A Unfortunately, the only thing not micro about microsurgery is the surgical cut. A 10-cm incision may be necessary as a large operating field is needed for the space to perform the delicate repairs. Adequate post-operative pain relief usually keeps the patient very comfortable. However, of late, tubal repairs can be done through the laparoscope but this is only performed by very skilled surgeons specially trained in the procedure.

Serial Killers and Bumps in the Dark

In developed countries, the main causes of death are similar. With improved standards of living, death from infectious diseases has declined whereas mortality from ischaemic heart disease, strokes and cancer has risen dramatically over the past decade. While conditions such as high blood pressure, high cholesterol level and diabetes do not kill, they predispose a person to heart disease and strokes. It has been said that an ounce of prevention is worth a ton of cure. As many of the illnesses are to some degree behaviour-dependant, it can be said that to a large extent, we are masters of our own destiny.

High blood pressure

Q What is high blood pressure?

A As a general rule, a woman has high blood pressure if her pressure taken at rest on two or more occasions, is 140/90 mm Hg or more.

Q How does hypertension cause heart attacks and strokes?

A A high blood pressure means that the heart has to pump harder against resistance. Also, the increased pressure damages the walls of the arteries and makes it easier for blood clots to form.

In both situations, a decrease in blood supply in increasingly active muscle predisposes a person to a heart attack. The increase in pressure also makes it more likely for blood vessels in the brain to burst or for blood clots to form in the damaged arteries, resulting in strokes.

Q How is high blood pressure treated?

A Early rises in blood pressure can be reversed by life-style changes. These include weight reduction, regular aerobic exercises and avoidance of stress. Once the high pressure has set in, life-long treatment with drugs is needed to prevent complications arising from the high blood pressure.

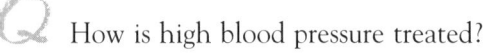

Diabetes

Q What is diabetes? What cause it?

A Diabetes is a disease characterized by raised blood sugar and fat levels. It is caused by the insufficient production or the diminished effect of the hormone insulin in the body. Insulin is produced by certain cells of the pancreas, an organ situated below the stomach.

Q How common is diabetes?

A Roughly 4 per cent of the general population above the age of 20 years suffer from diabetes. The distressing part is that these figures are rising, owing to unhealthy lifestyles.

Q What is the function of insulin?

A Food that is eaten is digested and absorbed into the blood stream as glucose. Insulin causes the glucose in the blood to enter into cells of the body, where it is converted and stored to be used later for energy. In a diabetic woman, the decreased amount or effect of insulin causes the blood glucose levels to rise and this is the main cause of the symptoms of diabetes.

Q How many types of diabetes are there?

A There are two types of diabetes. Juvenile or insulin-dependant diabetes usually affects those below the age of 40 years while non-insulin-dependant or adult-onset diabetes affects those above 40 years.

Q Who is at risk of developing diabetes?

A Diabetes is more common in overweight people and those above the age of 40. Smokers have a higher chance of developing diabetes. Family history is highly significant as well. If one parent has diabetes, then the chances of a person developing diabetes are higher. If both parents are diabetic, then the chances are even higher. In Asia, Indians suffer a higher incidence of diabetes compared to the Malays or the Chinese.

Q What are the symptoms of diabetes?

A In insulin-dependant diabetes, the woman usually complains of nausea and vomiting, extreme thirst and frequent urination. There is also tiredness, irritability and weight loss despite extreme hunger. Women with non-insulin-dependant diabetes often complain of thirst and frequent urination, unexplained weight loss, impaired healing of wounds and fungal infections of the genital area. Tiredness, irritability and blurred vision may occur at a later stage.

Q How is diabetes treated?

A For insulin-dependant diabetes, daily insulin injections are necessary as the pancreas does not produce sufficient insulin. Proper diet and exercise help keep the dosages low and facilitate the proper control of blood sugar levels. Non-insulin-dependant diabetes can often be controlled by exercise and diet alone. However, certain cases would require oral tablets which help stimulate the pancreas to produce more insulin or to enhance the effects of existing insulin.

Q What are the complications of diabetes?

A Uncontrolled diabetes causes major health problems because a persistently high blood sugar level damages blood vessels throughout the body. This results in impaired blood supply to the eyes, kidneys and nerves. Blindness, high blood pressure, kidney failure, heart disease and strokes may result. In severe cases, the nerves of the hands and feet lose their function and the woman may injure her extremities without realizing it. Poor wound healing compounds the problem and if left untreated, gangrene sets in and amputation of limbs may be necessary.

Q Is there a cure for diabetes?

A At present, as in the case with hypertension, there is no cure and lifelong treatment is required. It is essential for diabetics to adhere strictly to treatment schedules as this will help prevent or delay the onset of complications and allow the diabetic woman to lead a normal life.

Q Can diabetes be prevented?

A At present, it is not possible to prevent insulin-dependant diabetes. On the other hand, non-insulin-dependant diabetes, can largely be prevented by avoiding obesity and by eating a healthy balanced diet. There should be a reduced consumption of sugar so sweetened drinks are best given a wide berth.

High cholesterol level

Q What is cholesterol? What should my cholesterol level be?

A Cholesterol is a fat-like substance which is produced by the body. A certain level of cholesterol is essential for normal function but too high a level causes blockage of the blood vessels of the heart and the brain, causing heart attacks and strokes. As a general rule, a total blood cholesterol level below 200 mg/ 100 ml (5.2 mmol/l) is desirable. The higher the level, the greater the risk.

Q I have a high cholesterol level. What foods should I avoid?

A A healthy diet does not mean total abstinence from certain foodstuffs; instead, it means a sensible modification of food intake. In general, to lower the blood cholesterol level, you should cut down on animal fat such as skin from chicken and duck and the fat from certain cuts of meat. Instead, choose lean meat. Prawns, crab, egg-yolk and offal such as liver, kidney, brain and intestines are high in cholesterol and should be eaten sparingly. Eat more beancurd, nuts, peas, dahl and low-fat cheese and drink more skimmed milk instead of full cream milk. Limit your intake of fresh cream cakes and ice-cream. Use corn or soya oil for cooking and avoid cooking with lard or ghee. Boil, steam, bake or stew your food instead of deep-frying it.

Heart disease

Q What is the function of the heart?

A The heart is a muscular organ which pumps blood to all parts of the body at the average rate of 72 beats per minute. In a normal life-span of 74 years, it does this 2 800 396 800 times. To enable the heart to do this, the coronary arteries supply blood rich in oxygen and nutrients to the heart muscles.

Q What is ischaemic heart disease?

A Ischaemic heart disease is the condition caused by the reduction of blood flow to the heart muscles. This happens when the arteries leading to the heart become narrow from fatty deposits accumulated over the years. This is called atherosclerosis and its effects range from no symptoms at all through mild chest pains on exertion (angina pectoris) to fatal heart attacks.

Q What brings about atherosclerosis?

A Atherosclerosis is a disease of aging and is aggravated by high blood cholesterol and fat levels, high blood pressure, diabetes, lack of aerobic exercise, smoking and stress.

Q What is the commonest symptom of ischaemic heart disease?

A Chest pain on exertion is the commonest symptom complained of. It is typically described as a pain or tightness of the centre or left side of the chest which may spread down the left arm or up the neck. This pain is called angina pectoris and typically lasts for only a few minutes and is relieved by rest. Sweating and dizziness may accompany the chest pain. In angina pectoris, there is a temporary deprivation of blood to the heart muscles but no permanent damage occurs.

Q How does angina pectoris differ from a heart attack?

A Angina pectoris is chest pain resulting from a decreased blood supply to the heart muscles during physical exertion. A heart attack (myocardial infarction), on the other hand, results from a complete blockage of the blood supply to a major part of the heart. Unlike angina pectoris, there is permanent damage to the heart muscles. This is a very serious condition and a third of patients suffering a heart attack die before medical help can reach them.

Q What are the symptoms of a heart attack?

A In a heart attack, the pain of angina is much worse. It is described as gripping and prolonged, and is not relieved by rest. There is usually accompanying sweating, nausea, vomiting and breathlessness.

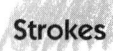

Strokes

Q   What is a stroke?

A   A stroke is a disabling condition caused by the interruption of the blood supply to a part of the brain, resulting in damage of brain tissue and consequent loss of function of the affected area. In severe cases, a stroke results in permanent disability, coma or death.

Q   What are the symptoms of a stroke?

A   The symptoms include weakness and paralysis, usually on one side of the body, often with loss of feeling on that side. There may be difficulty in swallowing, speaking or understanding as well as loss of concentration and memory. The patient also loses control of bladder and bowel functions, exhibits inappropriate behaviour such as crying or laughing at the wrong time and experiences moods of depression and anger.

Q   What causes a stroke?

A   A stroke occurs when an artery narrowed by atherosclerosis becomes blocked by a blood clot or bursts and causes bleeding into the adjacent areas of the brain. The latter situation usually occurs as a result of high blood pressure, injuries to the head, or from weakness of the wall of the artery (aneurysm) which may be present from birth. Sometimes a stroke is caused by a sustained contraction of the muscular wall of the artery (spasm) or from compression of the artery by a tumour.

Q Are there any warning signs before a stroke?

A Before the development of a full-blown stroke, there are often warning signs. These include temporary dizziness, fainting with numbness, and weakness or loss of sensation in one arm, leg or side of the face. There may be sudden unexplained headaches with blurring of vision and difficulty in speaking and slurring of speech.

Q What should we do if there are warning signs of a stroke or a heart attack?

A Warning signs, no matter how mild, should not be ignored as prompt medical attention can be life-saving. Do not drive to the hospital. Instead, call for help or the ambulance. While waiting for help to arrive, unlock the door and rest quietly on your side.

Q How can we prevent the development of ischaemic heart disease or a stroke?

A A balanced healthy life-style is paramount in preventing the onset of ischaemic heart disease or a stroke. This includes watching your diet to keep the cholesterol and triglyceride levels down, exercising regularly and giving up smoking. Periodic medical examinations are also important so that diseases like high blood pressure and diabetes can be detected early and treated.

Cancer of the colon

Q What is cancer of the colon?

A Cancer of the colon is a malignancy arising in the large intestines. It is getting increasingly common in developed countries and dietary factors are believed to be a major cause.

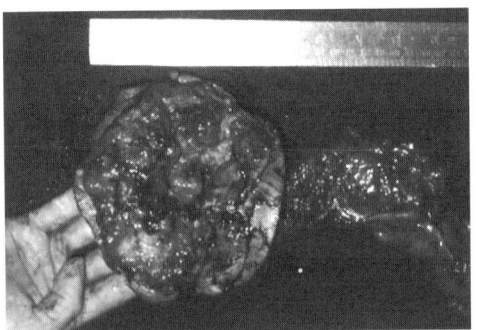

The large growth is the cancerous part of the colon.

Q What are the risk factors associated with cancer of the colon?

A About 90 per cent of cases occur with no family history and for these dietary factors are largely to blame. A diet high in red meat, animal fat and refined sugar, and low in fibre, coupled with a lack of vitamins C and A is believed to contribute to the development of cancer of the colon. In the remaining 10 per cent there is a family history of multiple polyps and/or cancer of the colon. These polyps have a tendency to turn malignant. This is sometimes associated with the so-called 'cancer-family syndrome' in which similar malignancies like that of the breast and stomach occur in the same family.

Q What are the symptoms of cancer of the colon?

A A large proportion of cancer of the large intestines arise from the rectum, especially the last 6 inches of it. In fact, a professor of surgery once said that we can diagnose 50 per cent of such cancers just by putting our finger into the rectum! In these cases, the patient commonly suffers from bleeding mixed with mucus. Cancers occurring higher up in the colon often produce a change in bowel habits or the feeling of incomplete emptying. Abdominal bloating, discomfort and tiredness from anaemia are other common complaints.

Q How can we prevent cancer of the large intestines?

A To some extent, this type of tumour can be prevented by consuming a diet rich in fibre and low in red meat and animal fat. Some, but not all, of the cancers can be detected by checking the stools periodically for small traces of blood. As the majority of bowel cancers arise from malignant change in a polyp, patients with a family history of such cancers should have a colonoscopy. It is advisable for high-risk patients to have a screening colonoscopy at 40 years. If the results are clear, then a repeat colonoscopy can be done once every 3 to 5 years thereafter.

Q What is a colonoscopy?

A In a colonoscopy a flexible black instrument the thickness of a finger is inserted through the anus to view the inside of the large intestine. Prior to the examination, the patient has to drink 2 to 3 litres of a laxative to clean out the bowels as stools would obscure the view of the internal lining of the large bowel. The patient is placed under mild sedation for the procedure and any polyps or abnormal features are removed for examination.

Breast cancer

Q   What is the commonest cancer in women?

A   The commonest cancer in women is breast cancer. It is estimated that every one in 20 women will develop cancer of the breast during some time in their lives.

Q   What are the signs of breast cancer?

A   Breast cancer is commonly detected as a hard lump under the skin of the breast or as a bloody discharge from the nipple. This lump is typically fixed to the underlying tissue and is therefore less mobile than a benign breast lump. There may also be enlarged lymph nodes under the armpits which appear as lumps. If the lump is neglected, the overlying skin may become puckered or ulcerated.

Q   Who is at risk of developing cancer of the breast?

A   Cancer of the breast tends to run in families. The risk of a woman developing breast cancer is higher than normal if her mother suffers from the disease. Having babies at a late age and having fewer babies increases the risk whereas having many babies and breast feeding them for prolonged periods protects a woman against the disease. Smoking and a high fat diet increases the risk of breast cancer.

Q What is the treatment for breast cancer?

A If the cancerous growth is less than 2 cm, preservation of the breast can be undertaken safely. The lump, together with a clear margin, is excised. If the growth is more extensive, the affected breast and the associated lymph nodes in the armpit are removed. In either case, the cancer is staged and if necessary, further treatment using radiotherapy or chemotherapy is carried out.

In patients with locally advanced breast cancer, chemotherapy is sometimes used before surgery to decrease the size of the tumour, making it easier for removal during the operation. Follow-up chemotherapy is usually required after surgery in such cases.

Hormone therapy can also be used in the early stages of breast cancer, especially if tests show the tumour to be sensitive to such treatment. Hormone therapy is also particularly useful in treating certain cases of advanced cancer which has spread to the bones and soft tissue.

Lung cancer

Q What are the symptoms of lung cancer?

A The common symptoms of lung cancer are a cough that does not go away, coughing up blood, a loss of appetite and weight loss. Sometimes, a lump appears at the base of the neck because of an enlarged lymph node.

Q   How can lung cancer be diagnosed?

A   Lung cancer can be diagnosed through a chest X-ray or CT scan and confirmed through a procedure called flexible bronchoscopy. Like hysteroscopy, bronchoscopy involves the introduction of a narrow flexible scope down the nose to the breathing tubes. Tissues can then be obtained for examination under the microscope.

Q   How is lung cancer treated?

A   Lung cancer is treated by surgery whenever possible. Unfortunately, this is not always possible if the tumour has spread or involves vital structures in the chest like the great vessels. Radiotherapy and sometimes chemotherapy are used.

The outlook for a patient with lung cancer is usually grim, because even with all the sophisticated equipment available today, less than 10 per cent of patients are cured of their disease. It is therefore very important to prevent this cancer by not smoking.

Q   How is smoking related to lung cancer?

A   Smoking is so far the most important risk factor in the development of lung cancer. Although only one in eight or ten people who smoke get lung cancer, this risk is many times more than in people who do not smoke. In certain parts of China, the incidence of lung cancer is one of the highest in the world. This is because of the additive effect of cigarette smoking to atmospheric pollution from factories and smoke from burning coal at homes for heating and cooking.

Ovarian cancer

Q What is ovarian cancer?

A Ovarian cancer is the malignancy occurring in one or both ovaries.

Q What are the risk factors of ovarian cancer?

A Ovarian cancer occurs more commonly in patients with infertility that does not respond to treatment and in women with fewer children. Use of the oral contraceptive pill and having many children protects women against ovarian cancer. Some researchers believe that excessive consumption of coffee and the liberal use of talcum powder on the genitalia is linked to the development of ovarian cancer.

Q What are the symptoms of ovarian cancer?

A Unlike the cervix, the ovary is an internal organ. Hence ovarian cancer tends to be ominously silent until an advanced stage. Common symptoms include abdominal swelling or discomfort, gastric or intestinal pains or bloating, weight loss, backache, problems with urination and abnormal vaginal bleeding.

Q What is the treatment for ovarian cancer?

A The mainstay of treatment for ovarian cancer is surgical removal of as much tumour tissue as possible and this involves removal of both ovaries, the uterus and the Fallopian tubes as well as the fatty apron attached to the large intestines (the omentum) as this may contain cancer cells. The cancer is staged at the time of surgery and if necessary, chemotherapy is given after the operation.

Q   When is chemotherapy used to treat ovarian cancer?

A   At the time of surgery, the cancer is staged. For advanced cancers, chemotherapy using combined drugs is usually used. Earlier stages of cancer may be divided into low-risk or high-risk groups. Those in the low-risk group merely require constant follow-up after surgery while those at higher risk of recurrence require platinum as a form of chemotherapy.

Q   What are the common side-effects of chemotherapy?

A   The side-effects vary with the drug administered. For example, the most common agent used in ovarian cancer, cisplatinum, causes nausea, vomiting and kidney dysfunction. To minimize the adverse effect of cisplatinum on the kidneys, adequate hydration in the form of intravenous fluids is given.

The side-effects of other drugs range from a drop in the white blood cell count to hair loss and a decrease in heart function. Some side-effects can be minimized through careful monitoring of the doses while others, such as hair loss, is only temporary.

Q   How can we decrease the mortality from ovarian cancer?

A   The survival of patients following surgical treatment largely depends on the extent or stage of the disease. The 5-year survival rate is 80 per cent for stage one cases, 50 per cent for stage two cases, 28 per cent for stage three cases and 9 per cent for stage four cases. Mortality from ovarian cancer can be reduced by early detection and treatment.

Cervical cancer

Q What is cervical cancer?

A Cervical cancer is cancer of the neck of the womb.

Q How common is cervical cancer?

A Apart from breast cancer, cervical cancer is the next most common cancer in the woman.

Q What is the difference between cervical cancer and ovarian cancer?

A Cervical cancer tends to produce symptoms at an earlier stage as the cervix is an external organ. On the other hand, ovarian cancer is usually silent in its early stages as the ovary is an internal organ. Also, screening for cervical cancer can be done using the relatively simple Pap smear and colposcopy. Early stages of enlarged ovaries, on the other hand, can only be detected via ultrasound scanning.

Q What is the cause of cervical cancer?

A Cancer of the cervix is actually a sexually transmitted disease. It tends to occur in women who started having sex at an early age, women who have had many sexual partners and women whose sexual partners are themselves promiscuous. These risks are further increased in women who smoke.

Use of the condom protects against cervical cancer. The secretions found behind the foreskin of the male penis is believed to play an important role in causing cervical cancer. Circumcised men have much less secretions on their penises. Studies have shown the incidence of cervical cancer to be lower for women in Muslim countries, where male circumcision takes place at the age of 12 years, and lowest of all in the Jews, for whom circumcision takes place at birth. Infection with the human papillomavirus and the *Herpes* virus are other factors which play a significant role in the development of cancer of the cervix.

Q How is cancer of the cervix diagnosed?

A Cancer of the cervix begins as abnormal changes (cervical dysplasia) many months or years before the development of actual cancer. This can be detected by the routine Pap smear complemented by colposcopy. Hence the importance of regular colposcopic examinations. Once there is cancer, the most common complaint is of irregular vaginal bleeding with increased discharge. The bleeding often takes place after sexual intercourse (postcoital bleeding) due to trauma of the cancer by the penis. The disease is confirmed by colposcopy and a biopsy of the most abnormal area. This not only confirms the diagnosis but also the depth of tumour penetration.

Once cancer of the cervix is diagnosed, it must be staged. This is done so that appropriate treatment can be carried out.

Q What does staging involve?

A Staging involves careful examination of the patient under anaesthesia. This includes a cystoscopy so that the extent of local spread of the disease can be ascertained. Cervical cancer is then classified into four stages. In stage one and early stage two, cancer of the cervix can be treated either by extensive surgery or by radiation treatment (radiotherapy). Late stage two and stages three and four cancers are treated by radiotherapy with or without chemotherapy.

Q What kind of surgery is done for cancer of the cervix?

A Surgery for cancer of the cervix is an extended form of a hysterectomy. The uterus, Fallopian tubes and a segment of the vagina are removed together with adjacent lymph nodes around the bladder, sides of the uterus and rectum. The ovaries are left intact.

Q What are the possible complications of this form of surgery?

A Bleeding and damage to adjacent structures like the ureter at the time of the operation are the main complications of this form of surgery, which is among the most extensive in the field of gynaecology. Later complications include problems with urination and passing motion as the nerve supply of the bladder and rectum may be damaged from the extensive surgery.

Q How is radiotherapy given?

A After staging, the patient is treated with radiotherapy 5 days a week for 5 weeks using a machine called a linear accelerator. The patient lies horizontally while X-ray beams are directed at the tissues of the pelvis for 2 minutes. The patient feels absolutely nothing during the procedure. After the 5 weeks of external radiotherapy are over, internal radiotherapy is given. A metal instrument is placed through the vagina and cervix into the body of the uterus and small pellets of radioactive material are inserted into the metal device. The patient then stays in hospital for 3 days, after which the metal instrument is removed and the patient goes home.

Q What are the complications of radiotherapy?

A Unlike the complications following surgery which are more immediate, the complications following radiotherapy appear later and may develop months or even years after the termination of treatment. This includes abdominal discomfort, diarrhoea, blood in the stools or urine and loss of appetite.

Q When is chemotherapy used to treat cervical cancer?

A This is used primarily for patients with recurrent cancer or when the cancer has spread, and when radiotherapy can no longer control the disease. Chemotherapy has not been proven to help in the earlier stages of the disease.

Cancer of the endometrium

Q What is cancer of the endometrium?

A This is a malignant change in the inner lining of the womb and is different from cancer of the cervix.

Q What causes cancer of the endometrium?

A High levels of the hormone oestrogen unbalanced by progesterone makes a woman more prone to cancer of the endometrium. This tumour occurs more commonly in obese women between the ages of 55 and 65 years. There is some link between these cancers and such factors as hypertension, diabetes and not having any children.

Q   What are the symptoms of cancer of the endometrium?

A   Irregular, heavy vaginal bleeding is the commonest sign. This bleeding does not respond to oral medication. Bleeding occurring after the menopause is very significant and any woman suffering from this must be examined to exclude cancer of the endometrium.

Q   What is the treatment for cancer of the endometrium?

A   Cancer of the endometrium is treated by surgical removal of the uterus, both ovaries and the Fallopian tubes. Radiotherapy and chemotherapy are employed in the treatment of advanced disease. Hormone therapy is also useful in patients with advanced disease.

Cancer of the vulva

Q   What is cancer of the vulva?

A   This is malignant change in the skin of the vulva.

Q   What causes cancer of the vulva?

A   Patients with vulval cancer tend to be above the age of 60 years, overweight, hypertensive and diabetic. There is an association between vulval cancer and infection with the human papillomavirus, herpes and syphilis.

Q What are the signs of vulval cancer?

A The commonest sign is a lump or itchiness over the vulva. There may be pain, bleeding, a burning sensation or ulceration of the vulva. In more advanced cases, there is a lump in the groin and the leg swells as the tumour spreads.

Q How is vulval cancer treated?

A Vulval cancer is treated by surgery to remove the affected tissue and the incision, interestingly, is in the shape of a butterfly. Lymph nodes in the groin are also removed. In extensive disease or recurrent cancer, radiotherapy is used.

Bumping off the killers

Having a family history of these diseases does not necessarily spell doom. There is plenty you can do to keep these killers at bay. On the other hand, not having a family history of these diseases is no cause for complacency either. The same sensible diets and life-styles are of equally great value in ensuring continued health and in improving health.

An apple (and more) a day ...

Q What is fibre? What does it do for me?

A You should certainly increase your intake of fruit and vegetables as these can only do you good. Fruits and vegetables are rich in fibre, a natural plant product which the body does not digest. Eating enough fibre helps in weight control, prevents constipation and lowers the blood cholesterol level. Importantly, it reduces the risk of heart disease, strokes, cancer of the large intestines and cancer of the breast.

Fibre in your diet can be increased painlessly by eating wholemeal bread, wholegrain cereals and unpolished rice daily. Finish each meal with a serving of fruit. The large variety available makes dessert very interesting and palatable. I have personally lowered my own cholesterol level from 260 mg/100 ml to 160 mg/100 ml in the space of 4 months by cutting down on red fatty meat and eating more fruits, vegetables, cereals and unpolished rice.

How not to go up in smoke

Q   How is smoking harmful?

A   Cigarette smoke contains more than 4 000 chemicals, of which 400 are poisonous and at least 40 can give rise to cancer. The poisonous substances include nicotine, which narrows arteries, raises the blood pressure and causes addiction, and tar, which is widely known to cause lung cancer. In addition, carbon monoxide reduces the amount of oxygen carried to the various tissues of the body like the brain and other organs like the heart. This makes it more likely for strokes and heart attacks to occur. In addition to causing lung cancer, heart attacks and strokes, smoking also causes severe damage to the lungs, leading to inflammation of the air passages of the lungs (bronchitis) and the break-down of the walls of the air sacs in the lungs (emphysema).

Q This sounds dreadful. Is there any other danger associated with smoking?

A Apart from the above, smokers have a higher incidence of high blood pressure, diabetes and ulcers of the stomach and the beginning of the small intestines (duodenum). It also causes impotence in men and infertility in women. Women who smoke are also more likely to suffer from brittle bones. In addition, smokers tend to have lowered stamina and suffer from frequent coughs and colds. They also have to live with ugly nicotine-stained nails and teeth, ashtray breath and wrinkled faces. The choice is really yours to make.

Q What about passive smoking?

A A large amount of exhaled smoke ends up floating in the air and is breathed in by people around the smoker. These innocent bystanders are then more likely to develop irritations of the eyes, nose and throat, a dry cough, heart attacks and even lung cancer. Young children are more susceptible and children of smoking parents are frequently troubled by coughs, colds, nose and throat infections as well as asthma. Furthermore, once ill, they also take a longer time to recover.

Q What should a smoker do?

A If not for her own sake, a smoker should stop smoking for the sake of her loved ones around her. The first step is to throw away all the cigarettes, ashtrays and lighters in the house and spend more time with non-smokers in smoke-free environments. Sucking a sweet initially may help you get over the urge to light up. Enlist the help of family and friends in your effort to stop smoking. By doing so, your body will begin to repair the damage and the risk of heart attacks, strokes and lung cancer will gradually fall. More importantly, the health of your loved ones will no longer be jeopardized.

A hearty work-out

Q   What are the benefits of exercise?

A   Regular exercise is not only enjoyable but beneficial to health. It aids in weight reduction, improves the flexibility of the joints, increases strength and stamina, relieves stress, reduces menstrual cramps and decreases the incidence of high blood pressure and diabetes.

Q   I would like to get started in an exercise programme. What should I do?

A   PLEASE CONSULT YOUR DOCTOR FIRST, ESPECIALLY IF YOU ARE OVERWEIGHT, OVER THE AGE OF 35 YEARS OR HAVE AN EXISTING MEDICAL PROBLEM. Once you have a clean bill of health, choose a game which you find enjoyable and which you can play with friends. This makes it more fun-filled and enjoyable. Also, start slowly with at least 10 minutes of warm-up stretching to avoid muscle or joint injuries. Initially, do not play games to the point of exhaustion. About 90 per cent of sports injuries occur during the first 5 minutes when the body has not warmed up yet, and the last 5 minutes, when reflexes are slower from fatigue.

Q   What is aerobic exercise?

A   Aerobic exercise is exercise which requires the muscles to work with an increased oxygen consumption. To be effective, aerobic exercise must be carried out 3 to 5 times a week. Each session should last 15 to 30 minutes and leave you perspiring and breathing deeply. It should raise your pulse rate to between 60 and 90 per cent of your maximum heart rate. The maximum heart rate is calculated as (210 – your age). Effective aerobic exercise is good for your heart and lungs.

Q   What are examples of aerobic exercises?

A   Examples of aerobic exercises include swimming, jogging, basketball, squash and badminton.

Q   What precautions should I take when exercising?

A   Wear comfortable well-padded shoes and light clothes that allow the sweat to evaporate. Drink plenty of water before, during and after exercising and remember to warm up before and cool down after the exercise. Importantly, do not exercise if you are feeling unwell or just recovering from the flu. Stop exercising immediately if you feel any chest pain, breathlessness or dizziness.

Q   I am too busy to exercise. What can I do?

A   You can exercise in the course of your daily routine. On the way to work, get off the bus one stop earlier and take that short walk to the office. Also, walk up the stairs instead of taking the lift.

When I first started walking up eight storeys to my clinic, I almost brought up my breakfast. However, after persevering, I can do it quite easily now and feel better for doing so. When in the office, stand up and stretch while talking on the telephone. If you are overweight, have a simple lunch of fruits and organize lunch time exercise sessions with your colleagues.

After a hard day's work, romp around with your children in the playground. Do not plonk yourself passively in front of the gogglebox after dinner but go for a walk with the family instead. You will find this a valuable time for family communication and interaction. On days when you do watch TV, try stretches and sit-ups at the same time.

De-stress or distress?

Q What is stress?

A When a woman cannot cope with the demands of daily living, she suffers from stress. Stress can arise from her home or work environment, her responsibilities, and the decisions she has to make. A little stress is good as it adds excitement and challenges to life. However, excessive stress or stress that overwhelms a woman is bad and can lead to poor health. Diseases such as high blood pressure, migraine, stomach ulcers, heart disease, depression, mental illness and even certain cancers are stress-related. Hence, it is essential to recognize when one is under stress and to be able to manage that stress.

Q How do I know if I am under stress?

A A woman who is highly stressed would have fast heartbeats, tense muscles, insomnia, poor appetite, headaches and diarrhoea. The woman also has a poor attention span and feels anxious and ill-tempered frequently. Menstrual irregularities are common in situations of high stress.

Q I feel stressed out. What can I do for immediate relief?

A Stress can be temporarily relieved by deep breathing, muscle relaxation and massaging of the neck and shoulders. These methods provide only temporarily relief and if you continue to feel stressed out, you need to analyse and deal with the cause.

Q So how do I manage stress in the long term?

A The first principle in stress management is to keep your goals in life realistic. Reaching for higher goals is fine, but reaching for the unattainable increases your stress level.

Equally important is effective time management. Learn to segment and budget you time. Running late for appointments and generally rushing around feeling that events are slipping beyond your control is bad for health.

Plan for and adjust to the changes in your life. Marriage, pregnancy, motherhood, career moves and moving house are all major milestones which require a period of adjustment. Stress arises if you still expect life to be the same as before.

Make informed decisions and consult the people who matter to you first if necessary. If on hindsight these decisions turn out to be mistakes, put them behind you and get on with life. Never cry over spilt milk as water under the bridge is just that – water under the bridge.

Above all, remember to be good to yourself. Give yourself some breathing space for your very own indulgences, as long as they are healthy and within your means.

 How important is mental attitude?

Be positive. Be happy and learn to laugh at yourself, at life and its lighter side. Learn to be content with what you have and make do with it.

Do not run away from problems but face them squarely. Share and vocalize your problems with your husband, close friend or religious leader. Sometimes the best advice comes from the most unlikely sources.

Above all, be kind, loving and respectful towards your husband and family. Respect your friends and treat the less fortunate well. Respect and care for a fellow human who is of little use to you is the true mark of greatness.

Learn to forgive as nobody is perfect. A harboured grudge is an extra 3-inch nail in your coffin.

Remember that what you carry up in your head and deep down in your heart colours your view of life and shapes your life. Being a woman should be a beautiful experience.

Appendix 1

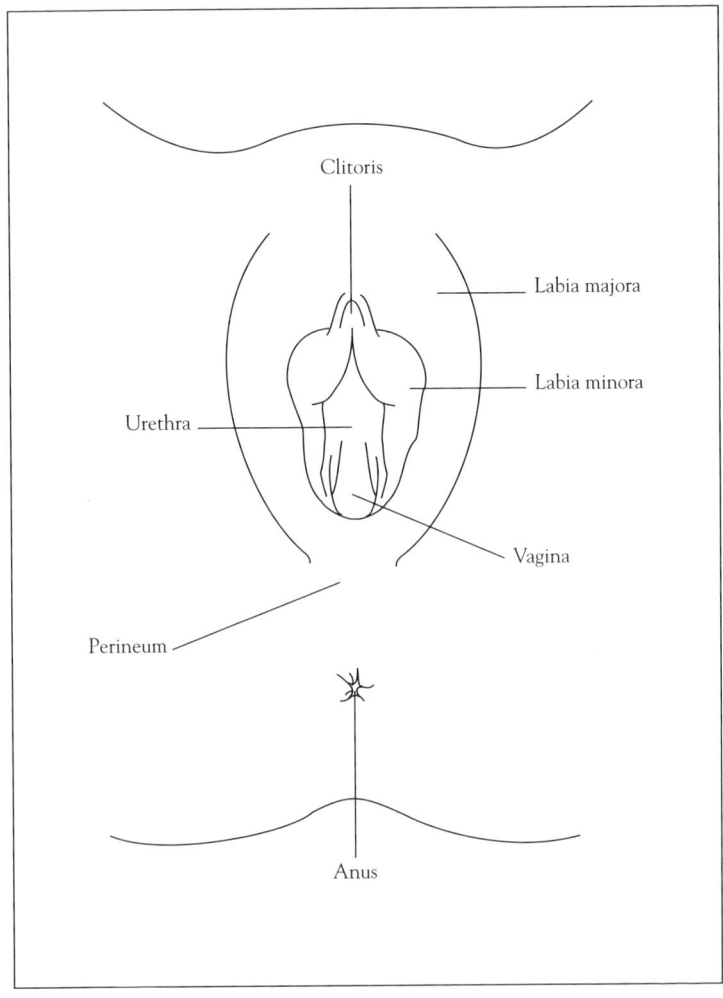

External genitalia

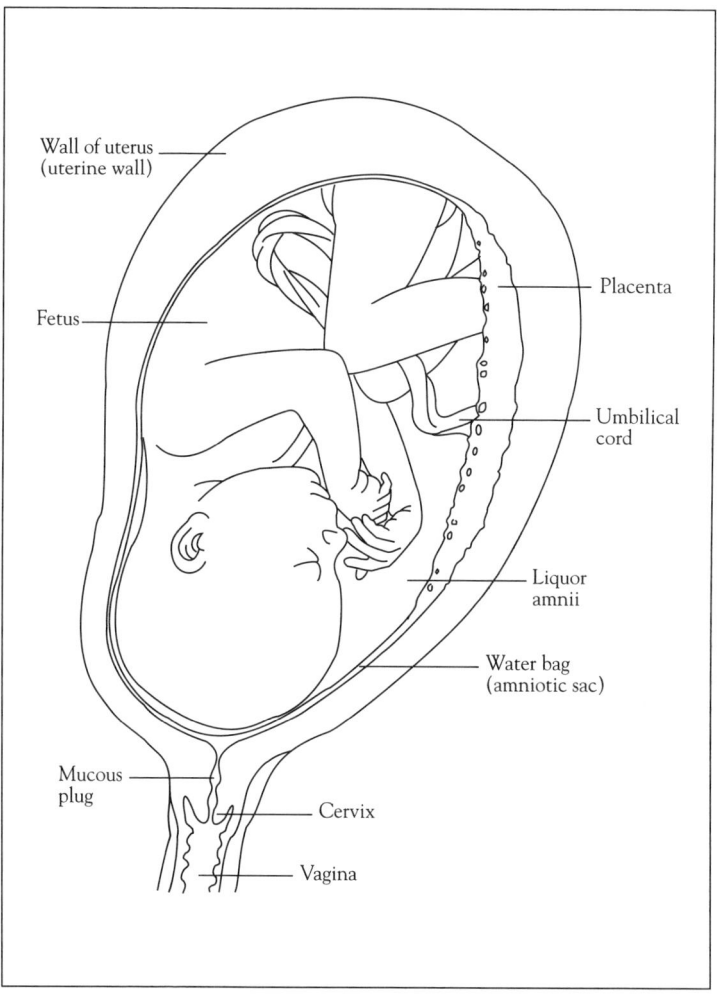

Wall of uterus
(uterine wall)

Placenta

Fetus

Umbilical
cord

Liquor
amnii

Water bag
(amniotic sac)

Mucous
plug

Cervix

Vagina

Cross-section of a womb with a term fetus

Index